Fitness And Exercise M

*Fitness success tips for mind-set developr,*
*planner creation*
*JimsHealthAndMuscle.com*
*Copyright © 2013 by JimsHealthAndMuscle.com*

Visit my blog for more expert advice on diet,
training, healthy recipes, motivation and more
jimshealthandmuscle.com
Please also "Like" at
Facebook.com/jimshealthandmuscle[1]
And Follow on Twitter:
@jimshm[2]#homeworkout

---

1. http://www.facebook.com/jimshealthandmuscle

2. https://twitter.com/jimsHM

FITNESS & EXERCISE MOTIVATION

**First edition. June 15, 2016.**

Written by James Atkinson.

# Table of Contents

Preface ...............................................................................1

GRAB YOUR BONUS ......................................................5

Introduction ........................................................................7

Why Take My Advice? ..........................................................9

Health Check ..................................................................... 11

The importance of motivation, self-motivation ................. 13

"Jim's Fitness Motivation Concept," .................................. 15

It starts with a reason ........................................................ 21

Mental Challenges............................................................. 27

Change............................................................................... 33

The Power Of Sustained Change ....................................... 39

Good and Bad Habits......................................................... 41

Sabotage/ Beware the "nay smith" ..................................... 47

Train Smart ....................................................................... 55

Excuses, Excuses ................................................................ 59

Visualisation ...................................................................... 63

Use The Force!.... Of Momentum. ..................................... 69

Speed Things Up................................................................ 73

Make It That Bit Easier...................................................... 75

You have to want and you have to own .............................. 77

Introduction to section 2 ................................................... 81

Step 1: Prep your chart ...................................................... 85

Step 2: Find your reason..................................................... 89

Step 3 mental robustness.................................................... 91

Step 4 change & habits ...................................................... 95

Step 5 Train Smart............................................................. 97

Reward yourself................................................................ 101

When it gets tough... And it will get tough. ..................... 103

Final Thoughts ................................................................ 105

# Preface

It's a cold dark day in October, the rain is lashing down with no signs of stopping; the wind is howling and the hope of a peaceful, warm summer's morning seems like worlds away.

From a warm cosy flat whilst sipping on a hot coffee, he stares out of the window at the torrential downpour and the stoic leafless trees that are being brutally assaulted by the relentless wind. He weighs up his options. He could sit back down, get another coffee on, maybe even make something nice to eat. It is Sunday morning, after all.

Or he could do what he had planned to do, get out there and make the journey to the gym on his bike to complete his last training session of the week. After some hesitation, he recognises that he has come too far to take the easy option and give it a miss. With a reluctance bought on by the thought of what he is about to endure, he puts on his training clothes, fills a bottle of water and heads down the stairs to his waiting transport.

The bike leans up against the shoe rack. It is an old and well-used thing that was given to him by a good friend a year or two ago. There are plenty of scuff marks on the frame and a fair few rust spots, but it has never let him down. At least this vital piece of kit would not be a target for thieves. With this in mind, he is aware of a smile on his face. He quickly puts on his waterproof coat, throws on his backpack, and opens the front door.

He wheels the bike out into the pouring rain and while holding the seat to steady the bike with one hand, he closes the door with his free hand.

"I'll see you soon" he mumbles to himself as he pulls the elastic draw strings of his hood a bit tighter around his neck. A few minutes later he is on his way to complete his training session. There is no turning back now, the hard part is over!

To some people, this little story may seem extreme and most would not need to ride a bike to the gym in the pouring rain to get their workout done, but the messages in this anecdote are at the heart of any fitness success story. If you can be the trainer or dieter that is serious enough about their goal to get out there and act with no excuses, you will be rewarded.

The easier it is for you to overcome stepping out of a comfortable environment into the pouring rain, choosing brown rice instead of white pasta or even starting your home workout routine, the easier it will be to reach, surpass, and maintain your fitness goals.

In this book, I will show you how.

Hi, I'm Jim, and yes, I am the guy who bikes to the gym in the rain and I have achieved a fair amount when it comes to developing my own fitness. But I would not say that I have a special gift or a secret that I used to give me an advantage over anyone else that would like to do the same.

Since my early teens I have been involved in some form of fitness training which has taken me from long distance running, bodybuilding competition, and I also served a number of years in the British army in an airborne unit (9 para sqn R.E).

As most people know, long distance running and bodybuilding competition are polar opposites when it comes to training routines and body condition, and I am not genetically built for either. So why is it that I can go further than most when it comes to reaching fitness potential? I believe that anyone can achieve great things in the fitness and fat loss game, there are no magic bullets, ultimate training routines or secret formulas to fitness and fat loss success.

The key is to become responsible enough to get yourself to where you are more than self-motivated enough to make the decision to step out into the cold and rain and make it happen!

In this book I will share my personal experience with some lessons learned that have been invaluable to me, along with some practical advice when it comes to overcoming the mental challenge that is at the crux of any fitness success story.

I base this advice on my personal experience of over twenty years in the health and fitness arena.

If you would like more useful fitness tips and advice, or you just want to stop by and say hi, here is my website:

# JimsHealthAndMuscle.com

I'd like to thank you for your purchase, and I know that you will get some great fitness results if you take on-board and act on the information that you read.

This book will give you many of the tools that you need to hit your fitness potential. This statement stands for all of my fitness books.

Before you start a new fitness routine, please check out my author page as there may be other titles that you can benefit from:

# James Atkinson (author page)

Il let you get stuck into the book now but I would just like to let you know that if you have any questions or comments, I would be more than happy to help you as these subjects are a passion of mine and have been for many years.

Big thanks to all of my family and friends that have been a huge influence on me. This has helped me to become the positive person that I am today.

Also, a special thanks to Tammy for supporting me through everything.

# GRAB YOUR BONUS

I strongly believe that anyone can get the fitness results that they want. It just takes a bit of consistency and work.

To help you get started, I have created another short eBook that you can download for free. You can use the information in this freebie in perfect synergy with this *Fitness and Exercise motivation* title.

The three main parts for fitness success are Mind-set/ planning, Exercise and diet.

You are about to read about the first step and I will always maintain that this is the most important. Without motivation and a plan, you won't get far!

But you also need knowledge of exercise and diet, and this is what the free eBook is all about.

The PDF holds some of my very own recipes. Everyone who knows me knows that I love my food! But living a healthy lifestyle means that some of the best foods are out of bounds...

Or are they?

I have messed around in the kitchen and created some great recipes (and some abominations, but fortunately for you, I will not share these) that are low in fat, low in sugar and high in quality nutritional value.

Exercise is also a big one, right! Well, I have taken care of this in the PDF eBook too. I've created a quick workout for beginners that highlights 7 of the most useful and versatile exercise movements that you can develop as you progress. These exercises are the bread and butter of most exercise routines and can serve you for the rest of your life.

As a 'thank you' for your interest in my book, I would like to offer you this PDF containing the quick home workout guide and the 7 healthy recipes to give you an extra boost and head start towards earning your fitness results!

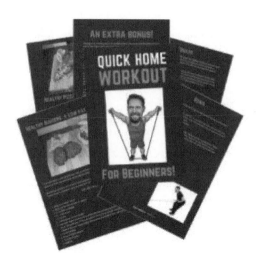

Simply click this link or copy the following URL into your web browser and let me know where to send them!

**https://jimshealthandmuscle.com/healthy-recipes-sign-up/**

Happy cooking!

# Introduction

When it comes to any type of fitness goal, whether the goal is fat loss for aesthetics and general health benefits or a more competitive goal such as sports conditioning, there is always a shared quality: Motivation.

Whatever your fitness goals happen to be, you will not get very far without the motivation that is required to realise your ambition. Sure! At the beginning of a fitness venture, everyone is motivated, but not everyone can sustain this motivation to see their fitness plans through to the end.

This book is all about starting from the very beginning of a fitness objective from the first thought. If you struggle to stick to a training routine, diet plan or have problems getting motivated when it comes to your health and fitness in any way, you should find this book useful.

There are a number of ways that you can keep yourself motivated, and there is a certain mind-set that you will need to adopt.

# Why Take My Advice?

Why should you take my advice? I have already given you a brief overview of my past experience, but if I were reading a book about health and fitness in order to glean solid advice, I would want to know how qualified the author was with as much details as possible. So for your information:

I am a qualified fitness coach (Trained through WABBA Qualifications in the UK). I am in my early thirties and have been at the sharp ends of several niches on the fitness spectrum.

During my time in the fitness game, I have been skinny and weak, fat, unfit and out of shape, a long-distance runner, passed para training and served a number of years in 9 parachute squadron Royal engineers in the British army and most recently been a competing bodybuilder.

Since December 2013 I have been writing fitness articles, books, training programmes and helped people around the world achieve their fitness goals. The power of the internet and the liberating evolution of self-publishing has enabled me to do this.

My thinking is that; it is all well and good deciding that you want to develop your fitness in one way or another; maybe you want to lose a whole lot of weight, or maybe you want to become a better runner, or maybe you even want to become a competing bodybuilder.

Once someone has decided that they want to change or work towards a fitness goal, the logical step for most is to find a fitness programme to follow and as you are probably aware, there is no shortage of these to choose from. In fact, this can be fairly confusing and a wrong decision can be an easy mistake to make.

Anyone that has read any of my other fitness books will know that I believe in getting real results from a training plan. This is why I put a huge focus on fitness for the long term and sustainable long term fitness results. I also believe that choosing a training plan is not the first step to take on your new fitness journey.

The first few steps that you should take are to create the foundations for the building of your fitness potential. If these foundations are as solid as they can be, your fitness goal, whether it be weight loss, muscle building or just general good health and wellbeing will be realised without the constant "yoyo training cycle" ie: Start a training plan or join a gym, give up a few weeks in, then rinse and repeat every six weeks or so until all hope is gone. The only thing this is good for is destroying motivation and an individual's self-belief.

Changing your body in any way is hard work! Most people will believe that the physical challenge of their project is the greatest test, but the mental challenges are by far and away the hardest part to overcome. In fact, I would go as far as saying that the overall mental challenges will equate to about 90% of the entire endeavour.

In essence, it is the mental challenges and lack of psychological preparation that are often the deciding factor in fitness success. Without the right mind-set, there is no chance that anyone can reach their potential.

This book is all about preparing for fitness success by first of all understanding the importance and the power of self-motivation and secondly by utilising a few practices that will help you create that solid foundation that you are to build your personal fitness success story from.

Before we jump in, I feel that it is worth enforcing the statement and mentioning again that getting results from any fitness routine or diet is hard work! So why make it even harder by not being prepared?

Get prepared! Plan and get yourself motivated! Use this as your starting point and don't skimp on this stage, take it seriously and your future-self will be extremely grateful that your past-self did such a good job at the beginning by laying those solid foundations.

# Health Check

Before you embark on any fitness programme, please consult your Doctor.

Do not exercise if you are unwell.

Stop if you feel pain and if the pain does not subside, then see your Doctor.

Do not exercise if you have taken alcohol or had a large meal in the last few hours.

If you are taking medication please check with your Doctor to make sure it is ok for you to exercise.

If you are in any doubt at all, please check with your Doctor first. It may be helpful to ask for a blood pressure, cholesterol and weight check. You can then have these read again in a few months after exercise to see the benefit.

# The importance of motivation, self-motivation

Everyone has seen great before and after shots of fitness success stories. Although many of these are "Photoshop at its best", there are also many that are true, real life endeavours. These images are often used to endorse a dietary supplement, a certain way of training, or a diet idea.

The one thing that is hardly ever mentioned is the hard work, self-motivation, and persistence that this individual has been able to sustain to achieve their results. It's all well and good getting hold of the best dietary supplements, diet plans, training facilities and the best workout routines that are available, but these things are nothing without the motivation to get out there, stick to your plan and see it through.

This is why I believe that you should take plenty of time to motivate yourself as an individual. The things that motivate you will not be the same as anyone else, this is personal, so you have to identify what is important enough to make you want to keep going until you get to where you want to be.

I believe that self-motivation is one of the most powerful skills that someone can learn. If you can motivate yourself enough to hit a good fitness goal, you can motivate yourself to do anything!

I learned to self-motivate subliminally. I left school at sixteen with below average grades after an academic struggle of nine years. I was pretty much written off when it came to chances of success "in the real world". I had low self-esteem and didn't feel that I would amount to much.

Although I would not get a career of any noteworthy standing, I was offered a job that paid good money for a sixteen-year-old with a contractor for British sugar. This was hard manual work, but I really was very grateful to Phil, the guy who gave me the job and by doing so, he had given me a chance.

Although I appreciated the fact that I had been given a job and was a valued employee, I really felt that there was more to life. It was a big world out there and I wanted to see it. The last thing that I wanted to do was spend my life in a nine-to-five job and stay in the cocoon of the town that I grew up in. So, with this in mind, it felt obvious for someone like me to look into joining the army.

After a lot of physical tests, aptitude testing, a bout of glandular fever and nearly two years later, I joined the army. During my time in the British army, I went on to pass P company (selection for airborne soldiers) and serve with 9 para squadron Royal Engineers.

After a four-year stint with 9 Squadron, I then became a fitness instructor and personal trainer.

If you fast forward a few more years, I am now making a living as a self-published fitness author. This may seem hard to believe when you look at the sixteen-year-old academic failure Jim with his low self-esteem and limited future. But it actually happened, and the lessons that I learned about self-motivation on my journey so far are the vital ingredients that made me believe that it was possible for anyone to achieve anything that they want to achieve.

# "Jim's Fitness Motivation Concept,"

One of the major observations in my time in the fitness industry is that there is a stage where motivation and drive to continue with the fitness endeavour is at a low point. More often than not, this stage is the breaking of most would be fitness success stories.

I have said to many of my past clients, readers, and training partners that the hardest part of a training routine or diet plan is the early stage, the stage where you make all of the changes, sacrifices and put in a whole lot of work and it seems like it is for nothing.

As a long-term fitness enthusiast, I understand this. I know that the work will pay off, but it is still a challenge for me to stay motivated. For the past ten years I have been in the weightlifting and bodybuilding game and in this time, if there were a few months where I needed to slow down slightly, I would never completely stop because I know how hard it is to start again. Instead, I would opt for a routine where I would maintain and just keep everything ticking over nicely rather than losing it all and starting from square one. To me, starting from square one is not something that I would like to do unless it was a last resort.

I am a veteran of fitness and have conditioned my body to the extreme, and if I decided to train for a specific goal, I would know that the work that I was doing would eventually pay off. But if it is this hard for someone like me, how hard is it for someone who is unfit, overweight with no real knowledge of training who is venturing into fitness for the first time?

It must be one of the toughest challenges that that person will attempt to overcome, and I imagine that to get through it they will need rock solid blind faith or a very strong understanding on how to create the mental robustness needed for this undertaking.

Being a visual guy myself, I find that having a graphical aid to help me understand a concept really goes a long way to help me comprehend an idea. So without further ado, behold "Jim's fitness motivation concept":

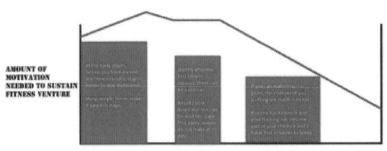

This is a very typical picture of the life cycle of a beginner to fitness. There are three stages here:

### The first stage:

Every single January, gyms and fitness establishments are getting ready to welcome new members who want to start the New Year with a fresh healthy lifestyle. Dave, Rob and Sarah all decide that this is the year that they will finally get in shape and earn the lean, toned body that they deserve.

Highly motivated, they all take advantage of the January offers and get the first month of their membership free and the joining fee waivered at their respective gyms.

Great stuff! They all hit the gym on January 1st and get their new fat burning routine sorted out by their new fitness instructors. The first session goes really well. And they are all looking forward to their lean future selves.

Rob and Sarah manage to stick to the new plan for the first three weeks, but Dave misses a few sessions because he decides to go straight home after work instead of hitting the gym on some of his training days. He is supposed to visit the gym three times per week on his way home from work.

Soon, it is the end of February and spring approaches! It has been almost six weeks since Dave, Rob and Sarah started their new fitness journey, Rob and Sarah are now seeing their first real set of fitness results. They are both stronger, have more energy, and can now actually see that their bodies have started to change. It has not been easy. They both doubted themselves at times and struggled through, but now it's starting to pay off. The results that Rob and Sarah have earned give them a huge surge of motivation, and it becomes easier not to miss a training session.

It has been two full weeks since Dave last visited the gym. Dave continued his pattern of missing the odd training session here and there until he lost motivation altogether and gave up. There will be a summer gym promotion soon Dave, or failing that there is a January 1st every year.

### The second stage

Although Rob and Sara are still training and have seen their first real set of fitness results, they are both struggling again. The initial weight loss and fitness results that they are earning are now starting to slow down, and the training sessions are sometimes becoming harder to get motivated for.

Sarah is happy with her results and starts to sit back on her Loral's a bit, she decides to drop one of her training sessions every week and just train harder in the two that she still completes.

Rob on the other hand decides to chat to a fitness instructor about mixing his training routine up a bit to spark a bit of new enthusiasm and see if he can get a further boost of fat loss.

### The third stage

It is now mid summer and Dave has re-joined the gym and is ready for another attempt. He took advantage of a summer offer that waivered the joining fee. Dave is familiar with the exercise routine that he was doing back in January, this fits in well with his lifestyle and he knows all of the exercise movements so he jumps right back into it and starts at the beginning again. The cycle starts again for Dave. Will he get past the first hurdle this time?

Sarah is getting ready for a summer holiday in Spain. She last visited the gym in April. The two training sessions per week soon turned into one and then dwindled to zero. Sarah managed to convince herself that her gym membership was not giving her value for money any longer, so it was cancelled.

Rob however still visits the gym, he now even works out more frequently. He has a good relationship with his trainer and has upped his game several times since he started back in January. Rob has lost a lot of body fat and he has also developed a good foundation of muscle, which is starting to give his physique a more athletic look.

As Rob has worked hard to achieve his goals and stuck with it through the initially unstable and doubtful times, he has seen some real results that prove that his hard work will pay off. From now on, it will become more and more unlikely that Rob will decide that he is going to stop training. Fitness and gym visits are now part of his everyday routine and therefore part of his lifestyle.

This is an example of the three most typical types of trainers that start a fitness venture. In my experience as a personal trainer, I can say that seven out of ten new recruits to fitness follow a similar path to Dave, two out of ten follow in Sarah's footsteps and only one in ten make it as far as Rob.

During my time spent as a passionate personal trainer, I found this frustrating and very disheartening. I wanted all of my clients to smash their fitness goals, surpass their highest expectations and be the inspiration of multitudes of others, but the longer that I was in the personal training game, the more it became apparent that it is really up to the individual to truly want to succeed.

You could have the best personal trainer in the world; you could spend hundreds of pounds or dollars a week and still not get the fitness results that you want if you are not able to self-motivate.

I had several clients that would pay me £25 per hour for training sessions. They would do this for months, staying inconsistent with the training routine that I set out for them and not taking the time that they were not in the gym seriously ie, bad diet and lifestyle. Each of these guys would be giving me hundreds of pounds of their hard earned money and getting nothing visible in return. This made me uncomfortable, and this moral dilemma of mine is the main reason that I don't do personal training sessions any longer.

I am now the author of several workout books, these range from £2.99 to £9.99. Now these books are fairly inexpensive and are based on the training concepts that I have used to get personal fitness results and results from my clients that were willing to put in the effort. I have also had plenty of readers contact me to let me know that they are progressing and hitting their fitness goals.

So, it confirms my theory that someone who is willing to do a bit of reading, learn to self-motivate whilst only spending £2.99 has a significantly better chance at hitting their fitness targets than someone that throws hundreds or even thousands at an expensive personal trainer hoping that this is the answer.

# It starts with a reason

Whenever anyone decides to take on a fitness venture, new diet, or healthy lifestyle change there is always a trigger. If there wasn't a reason to do this, why would it even cross your mind?

Most people who decide that they want to start a physical training routine or healthy diet will want to do this because of the way they feel. It might be that they feel overweight and unattractive, and when they look at themselves, they don't like what they see. On the other hand, it might be that they are training for a sporting event and changes have to be made.

If you are looking to start a new fitness regime, whether you have done nothing physical for thirty years or you have decided that you want to change the condition of your body in any way after a lifetime of training using limited methods, there is always a reason.

Most people, including myself in the past, overlook this extremely powerful tool by having a "subliminal reason" i.e. they don't know exactly what their reason is and this can really weaken the success chance of the fitness endeavour.

When I look back on my own personal experience, now I know how to identify my reasons for doing things, I can explain my reasoning for the big choices that I made now. But at some points in my life, I know could not.

I was in my late twenties when I first started utilising this tool, and it was someone else that set me on this way of thinking. I had been into bodybuilding in a big way since I left the army several years earlier, and I had wanted to compete in a bodybuilding show for the last few years.

I was speaking to a work colleague when we were on a break one day whilst showing him some pictures of some of the guys that trained at my gym that had already competed in bodybuilding shows. My work colleague was not someone that had the slightest interest in fitness or physical training, so I should have probably been chatting to him about something that we had a mutual interest in. But when someone has a passion for their goals or hobbies, they tend to want to share it with everyone and I had gone down this rabbit hole.

As he flicked through the picture gallery on my phone, you could follow his thought process by looking at his face. The subjects of these photographs were all men wearing nothing but a set of extra small posing trunks, they were smeared in deep dark fake tans with hard lean muscular physiques and to top it off, they were all striking some kind of "show off" pose.

As he handed my phone back to me, with a grimace on his face he said "Why do you want to look like that?"

In my infinite wisdom I answered in my typical light-hearted style with, "Chicks dig muscles, don't they?"

Although my answer didn't do a lot for the reputation of the bodybuilding community, it was no doubt the kind of answer that my colleague had come to expect of me as I am a bit of a joker, anyway. It was obvious that he wasn't that impressed with my plans and I felt like the time spent on the subject had come to an end so we steered the conversation in another direction.

On my way home from work that night when I had plenty of thinking time in my car, I thought about his question again.

"Why do you want to look like that?"

Now I was alone with my thoughts, I could be perfectly honest with myself without being scrutinised by anyone but yours truly. So, what were the real reasons?

As I made the forty-five minute car journey home, I set about questioning myself and searching to find the real reasons that I wanted to do a bodybuilding show. Most people don't want to do this kind of thing, so there must be something that had caused me to want to take up the challenge?

After being brutally honest with myself and facing the potentially humiliating truth, I came up with the real reasons. I was able to identify that wanting to compete in a bodybuilding show was a progression from overcoming an inferiority complex that I had when I was in my younger, more influential years and a need for the physical and mental challenge.

But If I had said that to my work colleague earlier he would have probably been left speechless as it would have been way out of character for me to confess such a thing. And in all fairness, earlier that day, I didn't know myself that that was the answer either.

When I was younger, I was always a small kid. I really wanted to be the Johna Lomu or Scott Gibbs on the rugby pitch and destroy my opponents with my awesome power, speed and bulk. When I watched these guys play rugby on the television for their respective countries, I would get goose bumps as they knocked other players down, broke out of multiple tackle attempts and carried the ball across the try line to lead their team to victory. But I would only ever be able to imagine what it felt like to be them. I was too small and weak to be anything but a liability on the rugby pitch, so I had to settle for being a substitute player. Until I found that I could work on my strength and size using a weight lifting routine!

Many years later, after overcoming many more challenges and learning some valuable lessons along the way that in turn shaped my personality and turned me into a different person altogether, I would jump at any opportunity to prove that I could overcome tough physical and mental challenges.

I hit bodybuilding hard and after a few years I actually looked like a bodybuilder, but to really reach my potential I would have to strip as much fat away as possible and the only real way to do this is with some solid accountability. What better way to put yourself under pressure to achieve a goal than to have a timescale and strong reason to accomplish that goal. If I were to commit to a bodybuilding competition, when the day of the competition came, I would be stood on a stage in nothing but a tight thong in front of several hundred people. Now if you were going to be doing that, you would really want to look your best!

On that drive home I found out a lot about myself and it was my true thoughts on a simple throw away question that my work college had put to me.

At that point I had committed to the bodybuilding competition, although this was months away, and I could pull out at any time, I wasn't going to, I would see it through and stand on the stage looking the best that I possibly could.

That now seemed to be the reason that would carry me to the finish line, but there were other powerful reasons that were working their magic too.

- I was in a job that was not suited to me and really needed a challenge outside of work
- I wanted to push myself to see how far I could go
- I didn't want to be an average joe who lifted weights and had a bit of size
- I didn't want to be the guy that said, "I thought about doing a bodybuilding show once,". I wanted to be the guy that said, "I did a bodybuilding show once, here's my trophy,"

- I wanted to add the bodybuilding competition to my "Have done" list
- I had been out of the army for several years and needed the challenge of hardship that goes with competition prep so I could taste the sweetest of sweet after the long months of sour when the competition was over. (This is an awesome feeling)
- I wanted an epic Facebook profile picture ☺

So as you can see, finding a powerful reason or number of reasons to take you to your own personal victories is not just a simple thought. To get the best out of this tool, you must delve deep into your soul and really try to hit the nail on the head. And the more honest that you can be with yourself, the more of an accurate truth you will find.

Remember that it is only you that knows your real reasons for wanting to change your fitness levels, so it pays to be as critical as you can be with yourself. This is how the most powerful reasons come to light.

If the reason isn't strong enough to drive the individual forward and force that person to their feet when the challenges of their goal brings them to their knees, then the reason isn't good enough! Everyone's reasons will be different and what one person might find ridiculous or even comical, this reason could be enough to push another person past the limits of even their own comprehension.

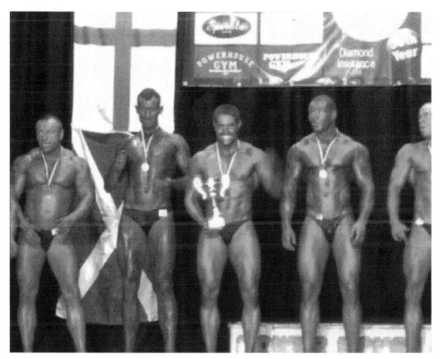

*"I did a bodybuilding show once, here's my trophy,"*

# Mental Challenges

When it comes to fitness training and making healthy lifestyle changes, most people will look at the physical aspect of the new undertaking as being the most challenging part that they will have to overcome.

But as mentioned earlier, this is a fair way from the truth. I can tell you that the mental challenges of any exercise routine or diet are by far and away the hardest part to overcome.

When it comes to dieting and training, I truly believe that the mental challenges when compared to that of the physical have a 90% share, leaving the physical challenges with a mere 10%.

In winter 2001, I was in the military. I had passed my basic army training and also finished my combat engineer training. During our basic training we had all been asked if we were interested in taking the tests to serve with 9 parachute squadron royal engineers or 59 independent commando Royal engineers.

At the early stage of our training, many of the guys put their names forward as there was a stigma attached to anyone who wore a maroon or green beret. These guys were (and still are) viewed as the hardest soldiers in the royal engineers who always get the opportunity to get in to the action first. These guys were viewed as highly professional machines that could be phased by nothing. Of course, when you are a recruit, you are very optimistic and pretty naïve and your outlook is "How hard can it be?" so probably about 60% of my intake put their names forward to be considered for the ranks of these "special forces" type guys.

By the middle of the second phase of our training, we were all asked the same question and this would be the point that anyone wanting to try out for 9 para squadron or 59 commandoes would have to officially sign up for it. At this point, everyone that had lasted the basic training and second phrase training so far had a pretty good idea of how hard it might actually be to pass these courses. Only three of us signed up for 9 Squadron.

When the day finally came, we had passed out as trained combat engineers and wore or blue berets with pride (later in my army career I would learn to call this a "crap hat"), all the recruits that passed were sent to different postings, some went north, some south and some to Germany. The three of us that had volunteered for 9 Squadron got posted right into the wolf pack in Aldershot to start the pre para selection process also known as "The beat up course".

For a new recruit and a "crap hat" 9 Squadron is a pretty hostile place to be. Previously we had only seen the odd one or two maroon berets walking around and these guys gave off plenty of attitude, but now all there was were maroon berets. Most of the guys didn't even acknowledge us, some quizzed us on who we were and what we were doing here in an all but friendly manner.

The beauty of this selection process is that the applicant can quit at any time and admit that this type of soldering is not for him. Until an airborne soldier passes the rigors of "P Company", completes his parachute jumps training and accepts his parachute wings, he is not obliged to stay.

On every training session during the beat up course, the squad of potential future airborne solders is followed by a Land rover. This is known as "The jack wagon". If an applicant is injured, passes out or just decides that he's had enough, he can jump on board, sit down and chill out. But if he gets on the Jack wagon willingly, it will be the end of his time with the airborne forces.

This fact makes it a lot easier for the applicants to throw in the towel. And coupled with the outrageously tough physical aspect of the course, it is under this psychological pressure that an applicant is tested on their mental robustness.

Early every morning of "the beat up course" about fifteen of us would form up in three ranks outside the barracks block, ready for the first training session of the day. It would be the three of us from my basic training intake (we were the newest to the military that were on the course) and the rest of the other applicants ranged from having served one or two years in the army and having ranks of lance corporal to even more experienced veterans of eight plus years and sporting ranks of Sargent.

The first training session of the day was always a straight up run or a weighted march/ run with boots and weapon. We would set off from the barracks and head towards the training area. These sessions would not be less than one hour thirty minutes. Anyone who has been to the training area in Aldershot will know that when I say "training area" I don't mean a simple running track. There were countless hills in this zone and a lot of these had names, "spiders", "sisters" and "flagstaff" to name a few. The ground was uneven and it had several different environments. There was loose rocky terrain, lots of potholed and puddled areas, and there was even a big stretch of sand that lived up to its name of "Long valley".

Every day, the training staff would try to break us mentally and physically and because the option of quitting was always there, it was not uncommon to be running with another applicant in the morning and come the afternoon, that guy was gone back to his unit never to be seen again.

On one such occasion we had set off as usual on our run. It was a particularly hard run that saw us starting at and maintaining a fast pace. It took us through hill sprint reps, firemen's carry hill reps, and it took us through our fair share of water and mud.

Everyone struggled through this training session, but there were a few that struggled especially. One guy in particular spent most of his time at the back of the squad and needed constant encouragement thought the session. He was last on all of the hill reps and carries, he regularly fell back and had to play catch up, but he stuck with it.

Even though this guy struggled physically through the training session more than most, was offered the comfort of the "Jack wagon" by the training staff repeatedly, he kept going. It is this quality of mental robustness that the para training staff are looking for.

As this training session was several weeks into the beat up course, we knew the area and knew when the session was finally coming to an end. We had all been pushed to our limits and were ready to get back to the showers and refuel for the next beating. When we were about 0.5 miles from the barracks the guy who had struggled so much now seemed to be finding his stride and had fallen in with the rest of us. Maybe the pace had slowed down slightly, or maybe the thought of finally finishing was spurring him on?

As the barracks front gates came in to view, I must admit that the site of steel mesh and barbed wire had not looked so inviting before. That was our finish line! It was only twenty feet away and the feeling of accomplishment was common through the squad. Everyone was running tight and together as one triumphant unit, including the guy who had struggled so much. Ten feet, five feet now, but the staff kept on running past the gate!

The session was not over. No more than ten feet past the gate, not only did the guy who had struggled so much earlier stop dead in his tracks, but other guys started to drop back too. The whole mood of the squad plummeted from high and triumphant to low and unhopeful.

The pace of the run did not change but moral received a devastating blow, turning the physical challenge into a mental and physiological battle that each man had to fight on his own. This was made even harder as one of the staff dropped back to the side of the now scattered squad and announced,

"Never assume that it's over and you'll get on a lot better on this course,"

This did affect me mentally, but I was able to overcome, and quickly accept that it wasn't over and managed not to outwardly show it. I stuck with the training staff as I had done through the training session and carried on.

We did not go back onto the training area, we merely ran to the next gate of the camp and finished at this one. It was about two hundred meters away. In that time we had lost two of the squad to the jack waggon.

To me this is a crying shame because it was a mental failure and not a physical one. So the guys that quit and changed their futures at this point were the victims of mental defeat rather than the expected physical failure.

These guys effectively shaped their futures by making a conscious decision to give up. It was the thought of the unknown that stopped them. If the staff had told them that we would just be going to the next gate, they would no doubt have flown through, even if they were asked to sprint to the gate, I believe they would not have had much of a problem in doing so.

For the sake of two hundred meters of the unknown, these guys would never earn a maroon beret. This was the first time that I realised that developing mental robustness can be the make or break of well laid out plans, especially with a fitness routine or diet plan.

I am aware that this is an extreme account of a mental challenge, but it is not as far away from the types of challenges a beginner to fitness may encounter as you might think. I learned many lessons from this one training session, but it is only recently that I have looked at it in more detail and broken it down that I can actually liken this single training experience to that of a long-term fitness or fat loss journey.

From my own personal experience I know the feeling of starting from the beginning of a fitness project and as I have mentioned in previous chapters of this book, I believe that this is the hardest part. The longer that you stick with it, the easier that it gets, but you have to be aware that it's not just a physical challenge, sometimes the mental challenges can prompt a devastating effect on your plans.

Another big take away is that when you think that it's hopeless, you should always keep going because you are probably a lot closer to achieving your goals than you think.

# Change

*"If you always do what you have always done, you will always be what you are right now,"*

Although routine and good habits are vital for any healthy lifestyle, sustainable diet or workout plan, a bad routine or can be hard to break. But if you are looking for serious results from a fitness venture, you must be willing to embrace change.

Most people are averse to change. This is normally because humans, like most other animals, are uncomfortable with the unknown.

It is easy to live in your own safe little bubble. If you have a nice structured life where you go to work every day, you know what time that you will be at home, you know that you will be able to pay your bills at the end of the month and you can pretty much predict what the foreseeable future will bring, you will be comfortable and the longer that you carry on along this path, the more comfortable you will become and the harder it will be to initiate a change of your own choosing.

For many people, this is the shape of things. Yes, there are possibilities of pay rises, yearly increases with some good employers but at the end of the day, the longer that you stay in a position; the harder it becomes to make the choice to change your trajectory. I am not saying that this is always a bad thing, it can be very rewarding for some people. I believe that this example of a comfort zone is the most universal.

When someone who has not been involved in any form of fitness before makes the decision to start a workout routine, diet or healthy lifestyle endeavour of any kind, they will have to make some drastic changes if they want to succeed and get the best results from their effort as they possibly can, and the longer that they have not been in the game for, the harder and more uncomfortable these changes are likely to be.

If you are the one who has been out of the fitness game for a long time, or this is the first time that you have decided to play, don't let the above statement put you off.

If you are aware that it is normal for the change aspect of this whole thing to be so tough, you will be better equipped to take on the challenges.

Eventually, if you stick to your new plan, the changes that you have made will become a part of your everyday routine and the metaphoric cement that is used to strengthen the habits of your new lifestyle will become stronger and stronger.

When I was dieting for my bodybuilding contest, I had to make many drastic changes as every bodybuilder should when they are preparing for a competition. I will admit that this is an extreme example and most people will not need to take it this far, but it is a great illustration to back up the point of this section of the book.

On the day before and leading up to the start of my precompetition diet, I was eating fairly healthily, not really looking at the quality of food that I was putting in to my body and I was eating a lot. I would basically eat high-protein foods regularly and it was great to add some chilli source, a bit of mayonnaise or some cheese in here and there. I would make a lasagne once per week for me and my girlfriend too. I would also eat the odd chocolate bar or cookie if the chance arose and it was always cheat night on Saturdays. Cheat night was and still is my favourite night of the week. My girlfriend and I order takeaway food and watch a movie. Cheat night also lives up to its name as this is our chance to eat chocolate, cakes and any other naughtiness.

So, one day I would look forward to every meal, find it easy to sit down and get stuck into the food that I had prepared and the next day I would be clock watching and dreading the next time that I had to eat. And if I were to stand on the stage come the day of the show and be a formidable contestant, I would need to stick to this lifestyle for the next twenty weeks without a single exception.

Every day from now until the contest, I would have to eat:

**Breakfast:** 100g rolled oats, 6 egg whites, 1 scoop whey protein

**Meal at 10:30:** 200g chicken breast 100g brown rice broccoli

**Lunch:** 200g chicken breast 100g brown rice broccoli

**Post workout:** Protein shake

**Evening meal:** 200g chicken breast 100g brown rice broccoli

**Before bed:** 100g brown rice, 6 egg whites, 1 scoop whey protein

As I had planned to compete in a bodybuilding contest for some time and had done plenty of research whilst training in a serious gym that was geared towards bodybuilding competition, I knew what to expect. But this was all theory until I was actually living it.

At the end of the first day, I was totally exhausted as I also had to up my training. I had to be out of the door at 5:30 every morning to do my cardio and be back with enough time to get my meals prepared, eat and shower before going to work. After my working day, I would have to go to the gym and do my hard resistance training before doing another thirty-minute cardio workout.

Between cooking, eating, working and training, there was little time for anything else and at the end of the first day I had doubts that anyone in the world could keep this up for twenty weeks.

This was not just a single change to contend with, it was a complete lifestyle change in one fell swoop. Nevertheless, I stuck with it and managed to get a good routine going. I started to become efficient at cooking, eating and washing up and with a slick system in place I could get this all done as efficiently and as painlessly as possible.

I even managed to negotiate a different break pattern at work with my boss. We were supposed to get a forty-five minute break for lunch and this did not work for me, so I put forward a request to change this to three fifteen minute breaks throughout the day so I could stay on track with my eating.

My boss agreed to this, but if she hadn't, I probably would have just walked out of the job. Although I made some good friends there, I hated that employment and my dream of bodybuilding was more important to me. It was actually a good thing that she agreed and I didn't leave as a few weeks later I was counting my penny collection in order to fund my new diet! But that's another story.

The changes that had to be made in order for me to achieve my goal were pretty punishing, but eventually I had adapted to create new systems and solid routines and it started to become the normal and easier to sustain.

Through the twenty weeks, I thought a whole lot about eating Chinese takeaway, pizza and I actually had many dreams about cheese burgers and chocolate bars. Even the thought of a nice chilli and fluffy white rice with some crusty bread and butter made me wish that this dieting insanity was all over.

The day of the competition came, I got ready, and my best friend drove me and my girlfriend to the contest venue. We drove in convoy with the two other guys that had also endured the previous twenty weeks' dieting to compete and a whole bunch of supports from our gym. It was a great day made better as we all returned with trophies.

From that evening, my heavy restrictions on food had been completely lifted and I had free rein to eat whatever I wanted. The night of the show was pretty much written off as I was exhausted, severely dehydrated and not in any state to enjoy a good meal. I did what I could and drank plenty of water, but ended up going to sleep at about 10:30pm. A few hours later and I had come to my senses, I woke up at around 3:30am with ideas of the potential food possibilities that lay at my mercy. I headed to the kitchen, and it began! I just started eating! Doritos, doughnuts, chocolate, cheese, peanut butter, I could even get a cappuccino on the go. This food was in the house because people had bought me it in the form of celebration gifts, and my sister had even made me a full hamper of "none bodybuilding food".

I did not go back to bed, I just kept eating. It was a Sunday and my dad had planned to do a barbeque for the family. There were all sorts here, all my favourites, and among this were the homemade cheese burgers that I had been dreaming of. This food had never tasted so good!

Although it was good to have a day where I could go at any kind of food with no regard for its nutritional content, I did not realise how dependent I had become on the diet and lifestyle that I had been living for the last twenty weeks. I had worked so hard to earn the body that I now had, that I didn't want to ruin it and go back to what I used to be. When you put in this amount of work with any project, you would not want to just throw it away and start again.

The first real struggle that I had was on my first day at work. I didn't have to do my cardio in the morning, cook egg whites, chicken, brown rice and broccoli. Sure, it was nice to get up an hour later, but it actually took me longer to make a few tuna salad sandwiches on rye bread, than it did to do my usual cooking, washing up and eating. Also in the first week back at work, I decided that I would go into the town and pick up some "normal lunch" like all of my other co-workers did on their forty-five minute lunch break. We were situated right on the doorstep of a busy town with plenty of choice when it came to food. But I really struggled to find somewhere that I wanted to get my lunch from. I didn't want to eat bread or flour based carbohydrates, I didn't really want to eat potatoes or other starchy products and I found myself totally lost when it came to lunch times at work. "A duck out of water" was never a better metaphor for my situation when it came to this change.

The extreme changes that I had made twenty weeks earlier that I had thought would be impossible for anyone to sustain had now become hard for me to move away from. Even now, three years after my bodybuilding contest, I still maintain some of the changes that I had to make in order to compete. There were many valuable lessons learned during this process for me and the power that sustained change can have on someone's lifestyle, not only in the health and fitness world but in every other aspect of their life can be staggering.

When you make changes that you know are for the best, have the conviction to keep it up and it will get easier to maintain and eventually become second nature.

# The Power Of Sustained Change

There is much to be said about the power and value of a sustained change when it comes to your fitness, diet and lifestyle choices.

If you start making constant small changes that affect your health, even if it is only one small change per week, you will be investing in your lifestyle in a positive way, much the same as you would if you invested your money in a compound interest scheme. (I'm not sure if such a thing exists these days, but the principals are there).

Albert Einstein said:

*"Compound interest is the greatest mathematical discovery of all time,"*

I am pretty sure that most people know the story of the two sons who get a choice of inheritance from their father on his death bed. But for those who don't, here is a quick version of it:

The choice is between one million pounds right away or a compound interest scheme starting at a penny and doubling every day for a month. With this second option, the son would also have to work his father's farm from dawn until dusk for no pay for thirty-one days; he would only be paid the compound interest with his first day of work, paying only one penny.

So the first son decides that he will take the one million pounds without much thought. He was not going to do a day's hard work for a single penny! He takes the one million pounds and gets to work on setting up his own new business.

The second son knows the value of compound interest, so he agrees to take the second option and gets to work on his father's farm.

By day five, the second son is exhausted; he has accumulated a grand total of £0.16p. Nearly a week's hard work and not even one pound to show for it. The first son who took the one million pounds has started to invest in his new business, he has treated himself to a few new personal things and has about £800,000 left to play with.

On day twenty the second son has spent a lot more on his new business, he has taken on some of his own staff to oversee the setup. He has now spent £600,000 leaving him with £400,000. This is still a good position provided that he has done everything right with his new business venture. While the first son has invested in a new business and has £400,00 in the bank at day twenty, the second son is still working hard on the farm and he only has £5,224.88p to show for it. He only has eleven days left, less than half of his time to make his final figure of inheritance.

It is not until the twenty eighth day that £671,088.64 doubles from the previous day to £1,342,177.28p that the second sons choice of inheritance option given to both sons by their father not only comes close to one million pounds but it shoots past it. But there is still a few days' work left for the second son. He works hard for these last three days and on the thirty-first day he finishes work on the farm for good and takes home £10,737,418.24p. This is nearly eleven times more than his brother took for his inheritance when he chose the first option that their father had given them.

If the second son had decided to take a few days off here and there during his months' work on the farm and forfeited that day's pay, he would have drastically affected his final sum of money. Just by skipping four days throughout his thirty-one-day working month, he would not even break one million pounds. The same applies to earning fitness results. You can see this working in the earlier chapter "JIM'S FITNESS MOTIVATION CONCEPT" in a fitness sense on poor Dave.

I love this story. I first heard it when I was at primary school. The fact that I even remember it from such an early age must mean that I was on board but, I really only noticed the true value when I saw the film "The happening" by Stephen King. In this film, the actor John Leguizamo quickly goes over it to try to stay focused or for some other reason while they are in a car........ Before it smashes into a tree and they all die.... But that part is not important.

When I saw this scene in the film, I immediately recalled the story from my primary school days and as I was much older, had a lot more life experience and so appreciated the meaning on another level. As I had spent a lot of time working hard for personal goals, many of which had been fitness related, I realised that the moral of this story fits perfectly into any fitness ambition as well as any other ambitions in life and it is never truer when it comes to the act of sustained small changes in relation to your lifestyle.

It is also worth considering that small incremental changes that are sustained and compounded over time can equally work in a negative way too.

# Good and Bad Habits

Habits come in several forms; some can be good and some bad. Every individual has an amount of both. Good habits and bad habits are one of the key culprits in everyone's state of health and fitness.

As mentioned in the closing paragraph of the last chapter;

"small incremental changes that are sustained and compounded over time can equally work in a negative way too."

This is where bad habits are to blame. Although it is true that many small changes that you make and develop into good habits will result in positive exponential fitness progression, it is also true that many small changes that result in developing bad habits will result in negative exponential health and fitness decline.

We all have habits and routines; these can be good or bad. But until you stop, think and identify what these are and what causes you to keep these habits going, you will find it a lot harder to stop them. You may not even know that you have a bad habit until you identify it.

Let's take smoking, for instance. Now this is clearly a bad habit and if you smoke, you know that you have a bad habit and it is not doing your health any favours. The thing with this kind of bad habit is that it will fit into your routine somewhere.

For example, every morning on your way to work, you light up a cigarette without even thinking about it, on your coffee break or lunch time and on the way back from work, you light up and puff away, it's just what you do.

Now this is all part of your routine, smoking all of those cigarettes adds up over time and the longer you do it, the deeper the roots and the more established the habit gets, and like an old oak tree, it will become very hard to remove.

If you are reading this and happen to be a smoker that struggles to quit and are thinking:

"What does a long term fitness freak know about how hard it is to quit smoking?"

Well, I have actually been a smoker and know all too well how this becomes part of a routine and in turn a negative habit. Yes, it is hard to stop smoking, but in my opinion, it is as hard as making any other lifestyle change. If you work to break the bad habit and the routine that comes with it whilst working on your mental robustness, you will overcome it.

Smoking is an obvious example of a bad habit as it is clear that inhaling hot black smoke with a ton of toxins in to your lungs to pollute them with tar whilst also poison your blood stream is not going to do you any favours at all. But there are many bad habits out there that are a hugely overlooked. Some can be very insidious and can be causing big disruptions to your health and fitness plans.

These days it seems that there are fewer smokers; in fact, it seems that it is actually a dying habit. But there are still some bad habits out there that can be addressed and stamped out to further escalate the fitness progression of a would be fitness achiever.

Most people who are looking to get into fitness for the first time, or even people that have been training for several years will be out to lower their body fat percentage whilst also developing muscle tone throughout their body or in specific areas that are particularly weak for that individual.

This is all well and good but it always prompts a sad sinking feeling in me when I see people working so hard to achieve their fitness goals, but they are overlooking or are simply unaware of some vital aspects that are holding them back. There are many examples of bad diet habits, but here is one that most people should be able to relate to:

Most if not all of the popular brands of fizzy drinks are completely useless and counterproductive to fitness, and specifically fat loss. These types of fizzy sugary drinks are packed with useless calories and rubbish, even most popular energy drinks that are associated with "pre workout energy" are counterproductive.

Personally, I have known people to drink several litres of these fizzy drinks every day. This has been a choice that they have made and subsequently it has formed a bad "drinking habit". The person in question was and probably still is very overweight and before I was as versed as I am now in the fitness and fat loss game, I believed that his genetics could play a big part in this and have a lot to answer to. I didn't know this guy very well; he was a work colleague that was based in a different office of one of my previous places of work, so I only saw him when he visited. As well as being hugely overweight, he was tall with it and I used to envy his bodybuilding potential. I always thought;

"If I had a body with that structure, I would be able to turn it into something awe-inspiring. I would no doubt be on the Mr Olympia and Arnold classic bodybuilding stage receiving cheques for $500,000 every time,"

Although this guy didn't have the slightest interest in diet and fitness I always wondered how he managed to get so overweight and so big, it must be diet right? But how could you manage to eat so many calories every day to keep this size on?

One day at work, there was a freak occasion where I was permitted to leave my office and go and help out in another department. As I entered the office space and walked among the work stations and cubicles of this new office I happened to glance at one workstation in particular where I noticed a familiar face. It was my work colleague that owned the body that I could have done so much with if it was gifted to me instead. Right away I noticed three, two litre bottles of fizzy drink sitting there. One of which was empty, and another was half full. Immediately, things started to make sense. It was obvious that this is a habit of my work colleague.

This snap shot of someone who clearly had a fizzy sugary drink problem provoked an instant curiosity within me and that night (after my training session of course) when I was at home, I grabbed a calculator and googled how many calories a typical can of fizzy drink contains. Knowing that these calories don't offer any valuable nutrition to the body I would find out how many useless calories were being consumed every time someone drank a full can.

I agree that this is not normal behaviour but it would answer a question that I could not answer for a while, so I had to do it.

It was pretty frightening! Typically, each can of fizzy drink contains 140 calories. Let's imagine that someone falls into the habit of drinking a single can every day with their lunch. At the end of the week, they will have effortlessly consumed 980 calories, just shy of 1000 calories. If you do this for a month, you will have managed to up your monthly calorie intake by nearly 4000 calories. After a year it would be 51100 calories! These calories do not come from useful nutrition like protein, vitamins, minerals and complex carbohydrates either, we are talking 51100 calories from refined sugar which is not useful for anything but weight gain and a development of poor health.

I will point out again that this is a single can of fizzy drink per day. On working this out I was shocked and had to do the maths several times before I was happy with it.

A single can of fizzy drink even as a treat or reward every day doesn't seem like a bad thing, but when you look at it through the eyes of a "useless calorie inspector" like myself, it shines a whole new light on it. If this is an everyday habit of yours and you are looking to lose body fat through new fitness and lifestyle choices and you drop it, or even cut it in half, you will instantly be better off.

There are many bad habits like this one working against many unaware, future fitness success stories and some that will eventually and also regrettably deny their host of this success.

If you don't want to fall victim to the insidious nature of some unidentified bad habits, you need to learn to first identify them.

It is always good to remember at this point that:

*"Your current state of health and fitness is a product of YOUR choices, actions and habits that YOU have developed,"*

**Bad habit triggers and substitutes**

There are parts of your daily routine that trigger your bad habits, such as coffee/ lunch breaks or car journeys. As you identify these, you will have a clearer picture of what you can do instead.

Let's say that every time you got into your car, you lit up a cigarette. You need to find a practical alternative to this.

By practical, I mean something you can do in the car instead. It's no good saying that you want to swap the cigarettes for tap dancing, probably not the best thing to do whilst driving your car to work.

I would invest in a "travel mug" you know, the ones with the screw-top lid that you can put into your cup holder in your car. I would make coffee or green tea in this before getting into my car and have that instead, and once you get used to this, if you want to quit coffee, you could swap this for chewing gum.

If you identify your bad habits and start to find healthier alternatives, your bad habits will become good habits.

Just imagine turning 10 bad habits that affect your health in a negative way into 10 good habits that affect your health in a positive way! Remember that this will not happen overnight and it is something that needs to start small. These small changes compounded over time will literally change your life.

There are many things you can do to break your habits. If you can just quit cold turkey, that's great. Do it! But there is the danger that this may be too harsh and you could crack under the pressure.

My argument is that if you are going to make a change that you want to be sustainable, you should do it with the view that it is a long term goal and a project that you can work on.

Be in it for the long term and you will see a lifetime of benefits.

# Sabotage/ Beware the "nay smith"

Everybody knows negative people, you may work with one, had an experience with one in the past or you may even be one yourself. If you are aware of the effect someone else's negativity can have on you and your fitness/ lifestyle goals, you will be able to identify the threat and guard against it.

There are two main types of negativity that can stop your fitness progression dead in its tracks or work on breaking it over time. Both of these are a real threat to your achievements.

The first is negativity from people who you don't care for, don't like or don't even know.

During my basic army training, I struggled with the fitness. I was by no means the weakest in the troop of new recruits, but I was definitely not the strongest. Cardio training and running had always been one of the weakest aspects of my fitness, and I would dread the cross-country running sessions when they reared their ugly head. At this point in my training, if I was told that a year from now I would be a machine when it came to this sort of thing, there is no way I or the corporal that was responsible for me would have believed it.

It was this corporal that first planted the seeds of doubt in my mind about my ambition to become an airborne soldier. Not long after the point in our training where we had just realised how hard p-company and para training might be and all but three had decided to take their names off the list, we were on a training exercise out in the woods somewhere in the south of England. This was probably only a few days' exercise, a week at most, and it would have been child's play compared to what I would become used to later on in my army career. But at the time, it seemed tough for all of us.

During these exercises in basic army training, there are unique opportunities to spend more time with the training staff. Whether it is by design or accident is unclear, but as you are out in the "wilderness" and working together, I suppose it makes sense that you will cross each other's paths a bit more.

The troop was split up into four eight man sections with a section commander (who was the training staff) as the man responsible for his section. The section commander was the guy who made the decisions, dished out the jobs along with any punishments. One night my section had an "admin period". This is a short break in duties so you have a chance to sort your kit out, clean your weapon, sort your feet out and eat. We all sat in the woods in a circle on top of our bergens (large back pack) and went about our admin. Unusually, our section commander had joined us. Voices were kept low as per standard operational procedures, we were in full darkness save for the odd glow of a burning hexamine block that was set into a small metal fold away stove, as some of the guys let their army rations heat up whilst changing their socks.

There was a general chit chat going on and the mood was fairly good. We broached such subjects as; the employment that we used to be in before we joined the army, our old lives and our first names (this got a lot of smiles as we never used first names and it was surprising to realise that we didn't even know the first names of some of the guys that we had spent nearly every waking minute with in the last eighteen weeks or so). Soon the conversation got onto P-company and parachute training. Our section commander had spent twelve years in the army so far and although he had never attempted the course himself, he knew plenty about it and he knew a few of the guys that were currently serving there. He explained how hard the course was and he talked about the "beat up course" before P-company itself and when I got the opportunity, I asked him a question:

"Corporal, do you think that I will pass?"

He looked at me and with not even the slightest hesitation he said,

"No,"

He shook his head and continued:

"From what I've seen so far, you don't really have a chance. Where is your shadow posting, Atkinson?"

As we were over halfway through our second phase of basic training, we had been given our first posting destinations. This is where we would effectively start our army career and it would be our home for the foreseeable future. As I had signed up to attempt P-company, I was assigned to Aldershot in the south of England to start the "beat up course" with 9 Squadron. But as there is no guarantee that a recruit and volunteer will even last five minutes on this course, he is given a "shadow posting". This meant that if I failed, got injured, or decided to retract my application for airborne forces training, I would have somewhere to go. My shadow posting was in Germany.

"It's Germany corporal" I said, feeling a more than a little bit de motivated.

He smiled slightly and nodded and he approvingly replied with

"Ah, you'll like it there, Atkinson. There's loads of drinking and German towns can be a lot of fun."

From this I understood that my section commander, a guy who was fitter than me, had a better understanding of army life and in my eyes was a successful soldier knew with 100% clarity that I was not going to pass P-company. I had never really liked the guy either, but I know this was by design. A recruit was not supposed to like his instructors.

With this kind of confirmation from my section commander, I started to think about retracting my application to attempt P-company. I would go to Germany and see how that panned out. After all, I could work on my fitness and reapply at any point in my career.

Although I "knew" now that I would not pass P-company, I didn't retract my application right away, I still had a few weeks to act on this and to be honest, the thought of backing out made me feel hollow.

If I had listened to my section commander and not even attempted P-company, I would be severely lacking in the self-development that came from this course and the few years that I spent with 9 Squadron as a result of passing it.

I believe that by not retracting my application and by not accepting my section commander's condemnation that I changed the course of my life for the better. I also believe that this decision was a major player not only in my future fitness but the foundation of mental robustness and the understanding of how to overcome any goal that you put your mind to.

Unfortunately, this type of sabotage has a lot to answer to. There is no doubt that it is responsible for countless fitness venture abandonments, and this is something that really annoys me.

Another classic example of this type of sabotage is the type of saboteur that will laugh at or make fun of a newcomer to fitness. People who are overweight and are carrying a lot of body fat are sometimes targets for this ridicule. It comes from people who have no business in voicing their opinions; they are thoughtless and don't understand the damage that they might cause. This type of incident can be extremely counterproductive. Especially to an individual who is in the early stages of their first fitness endeavour.

If you have been in this situation, experience this in the future or if the fear of this kind of thing is holding you back and actually stopping you from taking the first step towards a fitness goal, you should bear this in mind; If you let this affect your ambition in any way, you are giving in to them and effectively letting them rob you of your achievements. Don't let anyone with this kind of inconsiderate nature take away your goal.

Being told that you can't or shouldn't achieve something by somebody you don't like or being an unwilling target for criticism by a random stranger is one thing that can cause self-doubt or in the worst case a total breakdown of the fitness goal at hand and is an obvious means of sabotage, but being advised in a friendly manner by someone that is close to you that you rely on is how sabotage gets in with its metaphoric cloak and dagger.

Have you ever really wanted to attempt something challenging or had a goal but decided that you could not attempt it because you aren't built for it, you are not intelligent enough for it or you believe that you are simply never going to be the type of person who could achieve the goal? I have, and I would be surprised if there is a single person out there that can say they haven't.

Your decision may have not actually been yours. It may have been another influence that stopped you in the most innocent of ways. This is something that I only became aware of recently, but I now realise that it is one of the most unnoticed saboteurs working away to hold you back and stop you from achieving.

Every day, you are influenced by your family and friends in one way or another. These guys have your back. They have your best intentions at heart, but sometimes they can actually hold you back. The clearest example of this that relates to the shared experience of myself and anyone who has ever had a standard school education is that at school you are taught that you should study hard, get good grades and then you will get a good job working for a stable employer. This is what I and certainly anyone else in my age group was conditioned into thinking.

Since I left school, I wanted to be a millionaire and have complete financial freedom, and I wanted to achieve this by doing something that I loved. The problem was that I was never an academic and was already being stereotyped by my educational body as mediocre at best.

Subliminally, I always knew that I could not achieve this by simply working for someone else, but I was always told that I needed to find a job to get the money coming in. And this is what I did. Every job that I have done bar the army has been on a low pay grade and would never have given me the freedom that I had wanted.

It was the lessons that I learned through my fitness achievements that finally made me believe that I could achieve what I wanted in other aspects of my life. If I could go from someone that could not run a mile and a half in fifteen minutes to someone who could run a marathon any day of the week and pass P-company, or if I could go from a skinny long-distance runner to a competing bodybuilder, why couldn't I achieve financial freedom? Surely, I managed to do all this through hard work. Why couldn't I change my life in other ways?

It took me until I was thirty years old to realise this, and even then I was told by some of my close family members that I should "try it" but not to give up my day job. This doesn't work for me. I know that if you want to achieve a fitness goal, you have to be fully committed to get the best results. So to me, this venture was no different.

One day in late 2012, I went to visit my father with a bit of news that he would find displeasing to say the least. He knew that I wanted to quit my current employment working a nine-to-five job that I hated but he had advised me to stick with it and work on building my other business part time until I started to earn enough money to live on. Then I should quit.

On first thought this appears to be sound advice and I took it on board. But it was only when I reflected on every fitness achievement that I had accomplished that I realised that this would not work for me. If I was to do it as per my father's advice, I would not be 100% committed and would not be prioritising my dreams. So I handed my notice in at work and started working on what I really wanted to do.

On this particular Sunday morning I sat down with my dad and said;

"Dad, what would you say if I had handed my notice in at work?"

I didn't really want to tell him as I had an idea as to how he would react. I even toyed with the idea of not telling him at all.

His reaction was close to what I was expecting. His happy mood drained and he answered with;

"I would be absolutely furious,"

Hearing this and seeing that I had disappointed my father was hard to just ignore. No one of sound mind with a supporting caring family wants to be a disappointment to their close family members or indeed let them down in any way. But as I was expecting the reaction, I was able to talk it through and help him come to terms with it.

If I had taken my father's advice, I would have really struggled to even start. Compared to most, I am a slow learner and there was a lot to self-teach. It was more than apparent to me that my current employment would have the potential to damage my chances of success or even eventually beat me into submission.

Although my father had my best interest at heart and he didn't want to see me struggling, give up a "secure job" or put all of my efforts into something that he may have seen as a bit of a pipe dream. He didn't realise that his advice could have cost me my chance at a better future.

In the month of December 2015, I almost trebled the income that I would have earned if I had stayed in my previous job and not go against my father's advice. It would have taken me three months to earn what I earned in a single month, and I had taken the ceiling off my earning potential to boot.

This is a good example of the type of sabotage that is innocent and to all intents and purposes is not meant to be malicious at all. In fact, it is meant to be the direct opposite. When it comes to fitness goals, if you find yourself in a position where this is happening, to yourself or someone in the circles that you move in, you should address it.

It may be that you are very overweight, never done a single exercise session in your life, but you would like to have a go at running a marathon. Everyone who knows you will know that you are not a fitness enthusiast and they probably won't be themselves so they will maybe joke with you about the fact that you are not built for running or maybe tell you that you should start with a smaller more realistic fitness goal.

Although it's a good idea to start small and work up, you can still have the ultimate goal of running a marathon on your ambition list, but you should not be influenced or convinced to "downscale" your ambitions based on someone else's opinion.

The most valuable take away from this chapter is to be aware of sabotage and work towards learning how to identify anything that has the potential to damage your progress. Whether this is a blatantly malicious verbal attack, something said in jest by a friend with no ill intention or a value that you have been raised on, some of these saboteurs can be absolutely devastating to your progress and ultimately your fitness dreams.

If you find yourself in this situation, you do not need to react with an explosive torrent of hate filled anger at your saboteur; you just need to be aware of what's happening. The last thing that you want to do is fall out with a close friend over such a thing, you could just explain this concept to them or point them towards this chapter. This may even cause them to become more encouraging to you, and in the end become an essential asset in your fitness success.

When all is said and done, who has the right to persuade another to put a ceiling on their potential, take away ambition and ultimately stop them from achieving fitness deeds or otherwise? No one.

# Train Smart

In the chapter "Good and Bad Habits" we looked at how your routine and your habits fit together like a nice jigsaw. They work together without you even noticing. Whether you like it or not, your routine will influence your habits and vice versa.

I truly believe that routine is a huge factor in your success with health, fitness and your whole lifestyle. If you have a solid daily routine that promotes a healthy lifestyle and you have good habits to match, you should have no problem in getting the results that you are after.

Having a good exercise routine is just a single piece of this puzzle, but without it, the puzzle will be far from complete.

If you have everything in place, and you have consistency with your training, diet and lifestyle, you will no doubt start to see the benefits. This is great! Make no mistake; this is where you want to be.

But there is another factor that can put the icing on the cake for you and make your efforts count for more. Having a good workout routine that you can work from can make all the difference.

I believe that there are several components that make up a good workout routine. These components will make the routine sustainable and help yield the best results. They are:

- Progression
- Time scale
- Planning

### Progression
I am not going to knock the countless celebrity fitness DVD's that always seem to flood the market, especially right after the Christmas period because they do have a place for people wanting to start a fitness venture and these types of one off training routines can be the start of great things for the right type of person. But in the vast majority of cases, these one off routines are short-lived and are missing a few components for long-term success.

Progression is vital for fitness results. When anyone first starts a fitness routine, it will be at a certain intensity, it will take a set amount of time, use several exercise movements, have a set amount of resistance and so on. Normally, this will be great for the first week or two if the exercise routine is consistently completed. But with the absence of exercise progression results can start to diminish, and when this happens, there is a knock on effect and motivation inevitably takes a hit. When we lose motivation with exercise, we all know what can happen.

Therefor it is important when deciding to take on a fitness challenge that you pick an exercise routine with some form of progression. You should look at the bigger picture and find something that is progressive in nature. Your new exercise routine should have at least three stages of advancement, so if you find an exercise plan that has a "Beginner", "Intermediate" and "advanced" option, this is a good start. It means that you have something to aspire to and you have scope for improvement.

**Timescale**

A timescale should not be underestimated. Let's imagine that you have gone down the road of following an exercise DVD bought out by your favourite celebrity. You follow the on-screen instruction for the forty-five minutes or hour that it plays for and after you feel like you have done a good workout. Great stuff. You feel good!

But where are the milestones set out for you to aim for? Where is the progression, how long will it take for you to get bored and where will it end?

This is why having a timescale is so important for long-term success. You should have a timeframe in mind from the start. I would advise that you plan to use a workout routine that does not have any progression for no more than four weeks. This applies to aerobic routines that do not have any form of variable i.e., no increase in resistance, intensity or workout length.

Another important thing about a timescale is that you can create an "End game". Buy this I mean you have a certain time scale to achieve a certain goal. The best example of an endgame in my experience was my bodybuilding competition. The bottom line was that I had twenty weeks to achieve a physique that would not embarrass me on a stage in front of several hundred people, and I actually had a specific date that I had to achieve this by.

Getting ready for a bodybuilding contest is one thing, but a timescale doesn't have to be that long and the endeavour doesn't have to be that extreme. A timescale of two weeks is better than nothing. If you set out to lose eight pounds in body fat in two weeks from today's date, you have a timescale and a goal. This is the kind of thing that should be employed by anyone that is serious about getting results from their fitness training.

Another good tip in using a timescale is to have a specific date in the future that you want to achieve your goal by. If you don't have a date, you can create one. Let's imagine that it's the beginning of April and you normally have a beach holiday in August. You could book your holiday now and you will have four months to train to look good on the beach. With this "end game" set, you can now work on smaller "sub timescales". You could now work on a small goal every week, like the loss of around four pounds of body fat, and have a weigh in on a specific day and time every week.

## Planning

Without sufficient time spent on the planning portion of achieving a fitness goal, you will struggle! Every success story can attribute the accomplishment to a plan of some form or another, and the more in-depth and robust the plan happens to be, the better the results.

Everything in this book is leading up to the creation of your own bespoke plan that will almost guarantee your success. It is no accident that section two takes up a big chunk of the percentage of this book; it is dedicated to the planning aspect of fitness and lifestyle change. I cannot stress enough how important the whole planning process is if you want to get real results that you can be proud of.

Section 2 will walk you through the creation of your very own blueprint that will become your solid foundation and go to reference guide that you will be able to call upon, tweak, tick off and ensure your progress throughout your endeavour.

If you have not got a plan, it's like starting a journey without knowing your destination.

# Excuses, Excuses

Everybody, myself included, can find a good excuse for not doing a training session or for not making good dietary choices. But there really are no excuses.

Way up in the top ranks of excuses, if not the #1 excuse is the lack of time for performing an exercise session/ routine or for making a decent healthy meal. But as mentioned before, there really are no excuses.

I am aware that this may make me sound like a bit of a diehard, old school army drill instructor with no empathy for anyone who doesn't give 110% but that could not be further from the truth. My experience has proven to me that there truly are no excuses. I have managed to stick to a diet and training routine through some hard times, and I would class myself as an average guy. I personally know someone who lost both legs and one of his arms in an explosion, and he managed to cycle from Paris to London. Feats such as this should really put things into perspective.

Let's say that the average person gets up at around six thirty am, gets ready for work, goes to the day job and is back home for around six pm. It would be reasonable to say that this person goes to bed at around ten pm.

Supposing that this is all true, it leaves four hours in the evening. Four hours is a long time and realistically, a ten o'clock bed time is fairly early, but let's stick to these timings. It is fair to say that an hour of the left over four hours could be taken up with cooking and eating, another hour could be spent doing household chores and another hour could be spent watching the television or playing computer games. This still leaves an hour. Maybe a workout could fit in here?

When looking at this example, it is more than fair to say that I have been conservative with the time that it takes to do things. Realistically, you are not going to get home from a full day at work and spend a full hour on household chores every day and if you were, I would imagine that you would be an organised person that is more than capable of multi-tasking so cooking at the same time would be no problem and to boot it would be a time saver.

The point here is not to say that everyone has a spare four hours at the end of each day, because in truth everyone has a different set of circumstances. Some people might have children, some might work a shift pattern, some might have a disability. The point is that it is you who needs to understand that if you want results from your efforts, you need to make the time. If it means that you have to get up an hour earlier or go to bed an hour later, or even utilising your lunch break at work, then you should do it. But in truth most people can find the time without making any significant sacrifices.

99% of excuses are self-inflicted, and if you can accept this, you will be in a better position to counter any such excuse. You may have looked at someone else that is in better physical condition than yourself and accredited their ability to achieve this condition to their circumstance:

- They don't work the same hours as me
- They don't have children
- They are younger than me
- They live near a gym
- They have more money to spend on better food than me
- They know more about fitness than me

The list goes on. But as mentioned before, everyone has a different set of circumstances

I am not ashamed to say that in the past, I have looked at others that had a better physique than me and had thoughts along these lines. But now I am not embarrassed to admit it because I understand that it is probably natural to have this mind-set. I also understand the old saying: "The grass is always greener on the other side" and this tells me that they have their own challenges and if I were on their side, these challenges might cause me to look back at where I was and find similar excuses as to why I would have it better if I were back where I started.

So if you see someone who is having the fitness success that you would like, it's probably not because they have it better than you, it's probably because they have worked hard to overcome their individual challenges and earn their results.

Maybe you know someone right now that you feel this way about, or maybe you will find yourself in this situation at a later date. If and when you get to this point, it would be good to remember the old "grass is always greener" saying and be encouraging towards the person that is doing a bit better than you are.

You may even learn from them by asking them about their routine. There could be things that they do that you haven't even thought of that would give you a boost or make things a bit easier on your side.

Everyone has heard that there are "no excuses" and you would probably imagine the phrase in a fitness context coming from an elite athlete or hard-core bodybuilder at the top of their game, but when it comes down to it, this is a basic lesson that should be understood and accepted from the very start of a fitness journey. If you are the guy or gal that has sat around on the sofa eating pizza for thirty years, it applies to you as much as it applies to the first person that crosses the finish line of the London marathon or the tour de France winner.

# Visualisation

If you can see yourself achieving a fitness goal or you can see yourself in the physical condition that you aspire to attain, then this will really help you on your way. Self-belief and visualisation can be a very powerful tool.

There are a lot of people that won't give credence to this aspect of self-made success, but I have first-hand experience of it and will always look at it as a vital ingredient to any achievement.

If you believe in yourself, and your cause, your belief will become your armour against the negative factors that are always present in the forging of a fitness achievement. The longer that you believe that you can be what you want to be, and the closer to your goal that you get, the more resilient your armour against this negativity and other hindering forces will become until it becomes impenetrable.

Visualisation was something that I believe I harnessed at an early age, but by all accounts I was unaware of the positive sway that this would have on my life. It is probably the biggest help that I get (even today) when I struggle with my self-belief.

Before I lifted my first set of dumbbells or challenged myself to run my first mile, I played rugby. Or to be more accurate, I went to a rugby club every Sunday and joined in with the training. My dad had watched England play rugby on the TV for as far back as I could remember, and my sister and I were bought up with this game as a default. It was good to spend time with my dad enjoying something that he was passionate about. It wasn't long before I also started to enjoy watching the rugby.

When I was about eleven or twelve, my dad took me to the local rugby club for my first ever training session. There was not a single person that I knew, and all the other boys had known their team mates in previous years. None of them were newcomers to the game either.

Before this training session I had never even picked up a rugby ball, I was not a sporty, outdoor kid, nor was I socially confident. It also didn't help that I was and still am a slow learner. So as you can imagine, it was an understatement to say that I was out of my comfort zone.

I hated this first training session and didn't want to go back. I dropped every ball that was passed to me to the point that my new team mates would prefer to take the tackle or fumble the ball themselves than pass it to me. I was always in the wrong place; I was wet, cold and very uncomfortable, mentally and physically. For the whole of my first season learning to playing rugby, my dad had to convince me to actually go and train every single Sunday morning. On match days, I would hope that I was a substitute and didn't have to get on the field because I would inevitably make a fool of myself and also let my side down. Luckily for me, my coaches were sensible enough to see things in the same light. But they would put me on the field every now and again as they must have wanted to keep me interested and "motivated".

I hated not knowing the rules of the game and not knowing what was going on. I probably looked like a hesitant, nervous clown that was predictably going to run the wrong way or cost the team points when I got a "chance to shine" on the field on match days.

As I am a slow learner, it took me a while to figure out that when I watched the rugby on TV with my dad, I could ask questions. I could watch what the England player that played in the same position that I was allocated to by my coaches was doing and maybe get some tips from him. After all, he did play for England, so that made him the best player for that position in the whole country. What better teacher could there be than this guy?

It turned out that this guy was called Rory Underwood and his position was Wing. He was fast, strong, and whenever the ball came to him, there was a good chance that he was going to put points on the board for England. It was apparent now that I was put in the same position as Rory Underwood, not because I was strong and fast and I was far from a top try scorer. It was because from his position I would be out of the way and therefore likely to see less of the game play and in turn would be less likely to ruin the chances for the rest of the team.

So from now on, Rory Underwood and my dad became my teachers. On the first day that I started taking a bigger interest in the rules and dynamics of the game, there was a "eureka moment" for me. It still makes me want to palm myself in the face and cringe when I found out that my age group only played on a half sized pitch, which meant that the posts and try line (where the guys on TV scored points) were to the side of us, so if I got the ball I would run across the pitch instead of moving forward. So I was basically Forrest Gump without the speed and sense of direction.

Now that things started to fall into place with rugby training, I had my two teachers, I knew which way to run, and things started to generally make more sense to me, I started to enjoy going to rugby. It was not long before I had Rory Underwood posters on my bedroom walls and was scoring some absolutely amazing tries for England in my back yard.... On my own.

It was at this point that the power of visualisation found me, and until fairly recently I was totally oblivious to the effect that it had on my achievements. I remember the first rugby match when I actually wanted to be on the pitch rather than shy away and nervously wait as a substitute for the call to join in. On this occasion, we only just had enough players to make up a team so I would be playing a full game, anyway.

At the start of the game, before both teams moved onto the pitch ready for kick off, I confirmed with the coaches where the try lines were, so I knew which way to run and where the boundaries were so I would not run off the pitch. When kick off came and that game started, in my eyes, it was the first time that a game that I was playing in resembled one that I had watched on TV. Although the full size pitch was only half the size, the goal posts had been substituted with small marking cones and the world class stadium and screaming crowds were swapped for an open field and a few dads smoking pipes, but the layout and orientation was now as I understood it. What really made it exciting was that I was stood where Rory Underwood would be stood if he were playing this game.

During this game, I wanted the ball, I could see the try line, and I wanted to do what Rory Underwood would do if I was him. Every time the ball came to me I would immediately imagine that I was on the full sized pitch, the few pipe smoking supporters were an excited crowd that jumped to their feet and started cheering me on with a communal roar of anticipation, they would erupt when I carried the ball over the try line and it would be glorious!

There were probably only a few occasions throughout the game where I actually got the ball and managed to gain some ground for the team, but there was one that I will never forget. I remember it as well as the conversation that I had with my biggest fan after the game, my dad.

At some time in the final quarter of the game, one of my team mates passed me the ball, the adrenaline surged, I was Rory Underwood again. I ran towards the try line. As soon as I had caught the ball, I and everyone else knew that I had a very real chance of scoring my first ever try. We were close to the line and I probably only had ten meters to run. My days of running in the wrong direction were over and the try line got closer and closer. From my right, I could see my opposite number closing in and heading towards me. When I was two or three meters away from the try line, he had caught me and had gripped my shirt. I felt myself being pulled towards the touch line (out-of-bounds area) but I carried on moving forward, a few more strides and I could dive for the try line and score. I did just that. The ball was over the line and I held it on the floor, the whistle blew, I heard clapping and some disappointed tones from the spectators.

Lying on the wet grass having carried the ball over the try line was an amazing feeling for a few seconds until I noticed that my legs were in touch (out of bounds) and the referee had not given the try. I had been pushed out, and the ball had technically gone dead before I scored the try, so it was at best a "good attempt". Some of the spectators voiced that I was actually in and the try should have been allowed but in the game of rugby, the referee's decision is respected.

After this, I didn't want the game to end, I just wanted another chance to be Rory Underwood and score for England.

After the game, I think that my dad was as excited as I was. He had a big smile on his face and the first thing he said was:

"That was a good game, you were so close there!"

Returning the smile and enthusiasm, I replied:

"Yeah, I know. I think that it should have been given though, do you?"

I asked with no shortage of optimism.

"I was stood right by it and saw your last two steps. First step, only the edge of your boot went out but the next step was your full boot, so close though, next time,"

My dad replied. It must have been a great feeling for him to see that I was finally enjoying playing this sport and that he wouldn't have to do the dance of convincing me to go and play rugby or train on a Sunday morning any more.

Things drastically changed with my rugby escapades for a few years after this, and it was a quick turn around too. One week I hated the whole environment, the cold, the wet and the irresolute feeling that I got when it fell to me to act in a game play situation.

It feels like a long time ago now but this was a clear turning point for me, not only in my sporting life but in valuable lesson learning that would help me out in later life.

After I had a reason to up my game back when I was younger; I didn't want to embarrass myself on the rugby pitch, I needed to find a way to actually bring the changes about, and it just so happened that I stumbled across the act of visualisation. I gleaned some knowledge from observing one of the best personalities in my topics field and I found Rory Underwood. When I watched him play rugby on the TV, I could imagine how he felt when he caught that ball and turned on his pace as he headed towards the try line. I could imagine how amazing it was to score for your country and to hear the roar of the crowd. This was something that I wanted.

It wasn't until I had visualised this that my outlook towards playing rugby changed, but when it did change, it was a very substantial change. There are a few lessons that I learned from this anecdote regarding fitness and achieving goals, but the most significant is the presence of visualisation and the positive power that it can have over someone's entire life. Of course, just because I imagined that I was playing rugby for England, it didn't mean that I got invited onto the England team, but it took me from one end of the scale to the other in terms of, appreciation for the game, physical, mental and social development which as a result enhanced my life considerably.

I believe that I have my dad to thank for this lesson. If he had given up on convincing me to go and play rugby at any of the many chances that he was given to do so, and left me in my comfort zone, it may have been years later that I utilised this phenomenon, knowingly or otherwise, if even at all.

I believe that there is a knock on effect from every important lesson that we learn and act on, be it subliminally or consciously, and this was one of the early lessons in my personal journey. I am certain that finding and using the power of visualisation was one of the first blocks of my characters foundation and from visualisation, my self-belief was born to its meek existence ready to be worked into another powerful tool that would be responsible for other leaps of faith later on in my life.

# Use The Force!.... Of Momentum.

Stick with it. It will pay off!

Have you ever watched The World's Strongest Man competition on TV? If you haven't, you are seriously missing out and you should certainly "YouTube it"!

The organisers come up with outrageous tests of strength and novel ideas that are different every time. Now I'm not going to tell you it's a good idea to go and start flipping cars down the street or start doing squats with a tractor tyre around your neck, but I will say there are some things here that relate to our topic.

In most contests, there is a pulling event. This event is "in true strongman style" outrageous!

To the mere mortal, this test will look impossible to even attempt. I remember one year the strongman contestants had to pull a truck along a fifty metre track. The measure of this event was the time it took the contestant to get the truck from a standing start to the point that it crossed the finish line. The contestant with the fastest time won the event.

Each contestant would get themselves ready in front of the enormous lump of metal on wheels by cracking their necks, rolling their shoulders and having the judges strap the huge machine that towered over them to the contestants harness.

When the starting gun was fired, the strongman put all of his energy, aggression and power into getting those massive wheels turning.

The truck just rocks a little at first, hardly worth all of that energy for such a small result, hey?

But the more the strong man stuck with it, the more this truck moved, from a slow rock to a very slow crawl, then a faster crawl, then it started to roll nicely, then an amazing turn of pace to the point that the strongman is actually jogging the truck across the finish line with half the effort he started out with!

So all you need to do is get yourself a truck and a harness and start going for runs with it strapped to you and you will be away!

Only kidding, the point I am trying to make is that the reason that the strongman ended up jogging over the finish line with a truck attached to him is the same reason that you need to stick with your new plans for diet, fitness, healthy living or muscle building.

Momentum! Once you have your momentum going, you will end up jogging your goal over the finish line, not dragging it around with you like a sack of potatoes.

Obviously you will not be dragging big trucks around and your progress will take longer for you to notice.

You are not doing this over several minutes; you are doing this over a longer period of time. So your progress will be harder to measure at the start.

Your progress is more like the magic penny; the results are not apparent right away.

Imagine you did have a huge sack of potatoes on your back that you have to take ever where you go, but if you stick to your training and diet plans, you get to take one of the potatoes out at the end of the week.

This is not great for the first several weeks and would probably feel like it wasn't worth doing, but understand that if you are consistent and you always get to take a potato out of the bag each week, you will eventually end up with an empty bag!

An important thing to know here is that if you lose your momentum, the results could be devastating.

Some of the strongmen who attempt the truck pull don't make it to the finish line, they lose momentum.

After they have used all of their energy to get the truck moving, as soon as they allow this truck to slow down, there is no going back, these guys are exhausted and to get this moving again would be impossible.

Pulling trucks and emptying potato sacks are very different in practice, but as demonstrated, the principle of achieving results in both examples is the same.

Just like the strongman and his truck, your momentum will turn up. The strongman got his momentum after he put all of his energy into getting that truck moving, once it was moving, it became easier to keep moving, but if he let up on the momentum, the truck would slow down and stop with the momentum also grinding to a halt.

If the momentum is lost, it would have to be kicked off again. This would take the same amount of energy to get going once again and for the strong man it is game over at this point.

Luckily for us, we do not need this kind of energy at the beginning, but we do need some to get the momentum going.

We do however need to start somewhere, and as I have mentioned more than once so far in this book, I believe the hardest part is at the starting point. Have a look again at *"Jim's Motivational fitness concept"*. The example of Dave and Rob shows the loss of momentum and the harnessing of momentum, respectively.

# Speed Things Up

We have looked at how a few small changes made to a routine or lifestyle can have a big difference over time. Hopefully I have convinced you that this will work as long as you stay focused and consistent.

I know it is hard enough getting started and staying consistent, but a lot of a little all goes to add up to a lot in the end. So what if you could just add that little bit more?

This tip is not for everyone, but it is worth taking on board. If you have decided to start to walk one mile per day as part of your new weight loss plan.

You could go out there and do your one mile, stop and do it again tomorrow. You would still get your results if you stayed consistent and you would be doing a great job.

However, if you decided on some days after you had done your 1 mile to do another ¼ of ½ mile on top of this you would be doing more than you planned and giving that little bit extra. Just remember that every time you put in more than you are supposed to that this extra effort will also add up to give you heightened results.

This concept is true in whatever you are doing. If you are doing a resistance programme and working with aerobic exercises using sets and reps - you may decide to do 2-4 reps extra per set.

This way you will be adding that little bit more effort on these sets, and this in turn will be boosting your results even more over time.

As you may know, I have been into lifting weights for a fair few years and for many of these years I considered myself a bodybuilder.

Like most other bodybuilders, I would try to get as many reps as I possibly can out whilst keeping my lifting form.

If I am training on my own, I may reach 10 reps and that is good. But if I had my training partner with me, he would be able to assist me with probably 2 more reps for each set.

Two more reps does not sound like a lot, but I would not have been able to get those two reps out without my training partner and I would have not been able to put this extra effort in.

If I achieve these extra 2 reps on every set, I will be doing a considerable amount more and my results will be better and be achieved more quickly.

You may therefore want to exercise with a training partner or "buddy" so that you can encourage one another.

Doing a little extra exercise every day will soon start to pay off. The opposite is true if you do damaging things often – no matter how small.

This works with your diet. My old colleague that had the fizzy drink problem peaked my interest into the amount of calories a single can of popular sugary drink would contain and the amount of calories that you would consume if you drank a single can every day for a year.

It is frightening to think that you would be putting in 51100 calories with no helpful nutritional value, so if you cut that single can of cola out altogether, you would have effectively burnt off this number of calories in one year without any huge effort. You will have saved yourself pounds and £££s!

If you are on a diet and plan to have a cheat day or you plan to have a small sugary treat every day. To put in that extra bit of effort, you could cheat less on your cheat day or have ½ a cheat day. Or you could not have a sugary treat at all on occasional days.

Remember that these seemingly small extras will all eventually add up for good and bad. So let's try to do the good ones.

# Make It That Bit Easier

Challenges are a good thing. If you are challenging yourself physically and challenging yourself with sticking to a new routine, you are developing your character as well as your fitness.

This does not mean that you have to squeeze in as many challenges and hardships that you can find to make it as hard as possible. You should focus on your goal and try to find things that will help you achieve that goal.

If we go back to the example of losing weight as our goal, there are things that we can do to help us along with this.

The first thing you can do is surround yourself with positive, encouraging people and people that believe in you.

This can be a very important step that is often overlooked and not identified as a helpful exercise, and in some cases without these positive people influencing your choices, you may never even try to reach a goal that you are capable of reaching.

You should also look for support from like-minded people. Join a weight loss club or gym. You could also join forums on the internet. Places like this will really help as you will be able to relate to other peoples progress, concerns and setbacks.

It is also a good idea to read about other people's success stories. If these guys can do it then what's stopping you?

A word of warning here though, if you read too much, you may be tempted to keep chopping and changing from one theory to another without giving the first idea a fair chance to work.

For example, you read about someone that has had great results from being on the "Atkins diet" and you do that for a week before reading another story about someone having great results with an "Intermittent fasting diet" and you give that a go for a week before reading something else you think you want to try.

I'm not a fan of crash diets anyway but you will see what I'm getting at here, get your plan and stick to it for at least six to eight weeks then you might want to tweak it a bit.

Consistency is the key!

# You have to want and you have to own

I have already talked about finding your reason for making lifestyle changes. Once you have decided this is what you want to do, you have to actually do it! We have all heard of the phrase "actions speak louder than words" well it has never been truer at this point.

If your bad lifestyle choices and habits are well established it will be so much harder to get up and start out with a new way of life.

Making the decision to get in shape, lose weight, become more healthy is the first step of your journey. The next step is in my opinion the hardest. This step is from the point that you start your new healthy routine to the point that you see your first results.

Like the son that took his father's farm job and started working for a penny on his first day that was covered in an earlier chapter, you will start with very small results, but compounded over time you will start to see some truly amazing changes. If you can understand this and find the will to keep going, you will not become the person who throws in the towel and decides to give up because for all of the work that you have put in you are not getting staggering results right away.

This will take time, so stick with it because once you see this magic working you will not look back and you are over the hardest part, you are on your way to the top of the mountain.

There are many excuses for missing training days or eating junk food when you should be eating healthy or training hard. I have probably heard all the excuses, and it is the one thing that frustrates me more than anything.

The bottom line is that there are no excuses. If you are determined to change, you will find the time, prepare the right food and be organised and focused on your goal.

Many people will point the finger when they have cheated or neglected aspects of their new health venture, but a game changing realisation is to own 100%.

"I didn't have time to prepare my healthy lunch today so I will grab some fast food instead,"

"I finished work later tonight so I will miss my training session for today,"

"I didn't have time to train this morning before work,"

Yeah, "The Time" gets a whole lot of grief from millions of people every day and I think that this is unfair. You can look at time as a great reliable friend because it is very consistent, it never changes and surprises you, it is always there and you can set your watch by it.

If you don't have time in the morning to prepare your healthy meals for the day, you can get up earlier, you can do it last thing at night. If you finish work later, you can still get home and do your training. The gym might be closed, but you can do some cardio outside or some bodyweight exercises. Once a good routine has been established, this will become far less of an issue.

A very important lesson in the midst of this lifestyle change, if not the most important thing you need to take away with you is that it is all down to you, you need to own your problems, take 100% responsibility and be 100% accountable for your actions. If you can understand this and put it into action, you will do very well. Remember;

*"IF YOU WANT TO DO, IT'S UP TO YOU!"*

# Section 2 Taking action

# Introduction to section 2

So far I have rambled on about some of the personal experiences and lessons that I have learned through my own fitness undertakings, but I also know from personal experience that reading stories and taking on information doesn't mean anything without turning the information into actions.

This is the hard part and as you have seen, the lack of planning and understanding can be the breaking of a fitness drive. So in this section, I have designed a chart for you to utilise and help you on your journey. Having a physical record of your ongoing plan to track your progress and help you stay focused is an extremely valuable tool that is hugely overlooked.

I have designed this so it is quick and easy to set up and it will take less than ten minutes per week to update. This chart will help you to personalise the subjects discussed in section one and further enforce their meanings. If you work through the subsequent exercises in this section, by the end of it you should have a clearer idea of where you stand, what might be holding you back, you will have a plan and a starting point and most importantly, you will be much better equipped and prepared to start and achieve your new fitness goals.

This part of the book is important. If you take this seriously and actually put pen to paper, it is a big step in the right direction. I love to hear that anyone that has read my books has taken the advice, acted on it and is on the way to earning their results.

The planning and preparation of a fitness ambition is a major player in its success rate so, lay the strong foundations and let's get building.

Most people's first step on a fitness journey will be to join a gym, buy an exercise routine book or other virtual training plan or even put their training shoes on and go for a run. But it will really help if you look at this part as the starting point. Take the time to plan. This is the first, true training session of your fitness journey!

Here is an example of the chart. I have used an instance of my "past self". As you are aware of my fitness background, my goals and the earlier struggles that I faced when it came to fitness, as explained in section one, this example may help you to more easily connect with the idea of creating a chart that is relevant to yourself.

When I was around fourteen years of age, rugby was my passion and I loved the game, but I was a slow developer among my peers. Physically, it seemed that I was about a year behind everyone else and at this age, that is a long way behind. This meant that I was smaller and weaker than the rest of the rugby team, and I would once again be a liability on the rugby pitch. I needed to get bigger and stronger if I wanted to play this game with my peers.

Logically, the best way to get bigger and stronger is to hit the gym and start lifting weights, eat more quality food, and this is exactly what I did. So if I were at this point again and I knew what I know now and furthermore, I decided to create a chart based on this book, the first week would look like this:

# SwapFat4Fit

**5 positive things that happened this week**

- Found someone to cook me... with weights
- Found a training partner
- Learned how to cook meatballs
- Was only late for school once
- Feeling positive about my plan

**Get bigger and stronger so I can play a great game of rugby!**

| week | Habit/change + Substitute | Training days | Reward |
|---|---|---|---|
| 1 | Train with weights 3 times per week | Mon, Wed, Fri | Cheat food on Sat night |
| 2 | Eat 4 balanced meals per day | Mon, Wed, Fri | Cheat food on Sat night |
| 3 | Drink a protein shake every day | Mon, Wed, Fri | Cheat food on Sat night |
| 4 | Sprint training once per week | Mon, Wed, Fri, Sat | Cheat food on Sat night |
| 5 | Practice catching for an hour per week | Mon, Wed, Fri, Sat, Sun | Cheat food on Sat night |
| 6 | Watch 1 pro rugby game per week | Mon, Wed, Fri, Sat, Sun | Cheat food on Sat night |
| 7 | | | |
| 8 | | | |
| 9 | | | |
| 10 | | | |
| 11 | | | |
| 12 | | | |
| 13 | | | |

# Step 1: Prep your chart

Your chart is going to be a creation that is unique and relevant to you. This is a piece of work that will be ongoing and will serve as a kind of elaborate diary that serves a purpose. As this is your own creation, please feel free to devise your own if you would prefer a better layout or you would like to add something to it.

If you don't have any ideas that will enhance this chart to fit in with your personal needs, by all means print this one off.

At this point I will tell you about a free resource that I have made that relates directly to this. Since writing this book I have had a lot of feedback from readers and I decided to create the ***"Home workout for beginners video course"***. As you probably know by now, I take motivation, planning and prep seriously and see this process as a vital part of anyone's fitness journey if they really wish to achieve their goals.

It's for this reason that I decided to add an in-depth module to the course – *"The planning and prep module"*! As you are reading this and have invested not only your money but your time in this book, I would love to share this with you.

The module is video based and is set out in five sections complete with an updated, downloadable PDF chart for you to print out. Just sit down with me and follow along. You can even grab a cup of tea while we work through and create your personal plan to fitness success together!

If this is something that you think is up your street, go to **YourFitnessSuccess.com**, sign up for the free trial and let's get started.

If you have any problems with the link, drop me an email, hit me up on the Facebook page and I'll do my best to sort you out with access.

With all that said, let's get back to the explanation in this book. In my chart example, there are seven features:

1. Reason for wanting to achieve the goal
2. 5 positive experiences that happened this week
3. A week counter to align several features on the chart (used to monitor progress)

4. Habits to change or changes to make and substitute (if any)
5. Training days
6. Visualisation aid *"pin visualisation aid here,"*
7. A reward Colum

- However you decide to obtain a physical version of your chart, make sure you have at least one copy and a template of it that you can easily duplicate. Make sure that you keep the template version of this chart in a safe place, which is easily accessible. The best thing to do is to have a bunch of these charts printed off so that when you fill one up, you can easily pin a new one over the top and carry on with no hassle.

- Once you have your chart, you need to find a suitable home for it. Ideally, the chart should be pinned up in a room in your house where you will see it frequently. The kitchen or bathroom tend to be good choices as they are normally easily accessible and they see the most activity. If you are following a home workout routine, you could put the chart in the room where you exercise. The idea is to have this chart somewhere where it will always be seen so it will be no good if you choose your attic or store room that you only visit once per month. When you have a good location for your chart, attach a pen with some string or just clip it on (you don't want to be searching for something to write with every time you need to fill it in). Finally, pin it up!

(On the following page, there is a blank chart that you may want to photocopy and blow up if you cannot get the direct download for whatever reason. You can even cut this out of the book if you have the paperback copy)

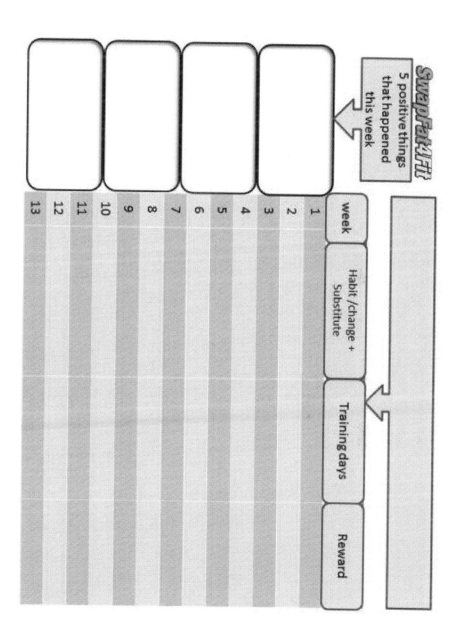

**SwapFatFit**

5 positive things that happened this week

| week | Habit /change + Substitute | Training days | Reward |
|------|---------------------------|---------------|--------|
| 1 | | | |
| 2 | | | |
| 3 | | | |
| 4 | | | |
| 5 | | | |
| 6 | | | |
| 7 | | | |
| 8 | | | |
| 9 | | | |
| 10 | | | |
| 11 | | | |
| 12 | | | |
| 13 | | | |

# Step 2: Find your reason

If you have a powerful reason, when things get tough, you can reflect on this and use it as a driving force.

When the time comes for you to define your reason/ reasons for wanting to achieve a certain fitness goal, as mentioned before, you should take it seriously and make sure that you set aside some time to dedicate to this important step. It may sound like a bit of a chore or even feel silly, but please have faith in this process; it will make all the difference. Follow these bullet points before moving on to step 3:

- Set aside at least fifteen minutes, where you are alone and in a place that you will not be interrupted.

- Sit down with a physical notepad and pen or even open a word document on your PC

- List all of the reasons that you would like to achieve your fitness goal. Remember to be honest with yourself. The more honest that you can be and the deeper that you can delve, the more powerful your reasons will be.

- If you are struggling, feel free to read the *"It starts with a reason"* chapter again, this may give you some ideas or inspiration.

- Once you have a powerful reason or a statement that encompasses several of your reasons for your fitness goal, fill in the space provided on your chart. Make it big, bold and colourful if you like. This needs to stand out.

- If you have decided to use the example chart that I have created, great! You will notice the space on there for your reason is fairly big and you may even want to put a visual aid in here to help too. You could use a photograph, quote or anything else that is significant to your reason..

# Step 3 mental robustness

Achieving fitness and fat loss goals is a mentally challenging game, and to win, you need to have a good resolve when it comes to mental robustness.

This planning process and the upkeep of your chart are actually working to develop your mental robustness. Although the development of mental robustness is something that grows as your fitness levels progress, there are a few exercises that you can do to actively help with the process.

For the purpose of this book and with the plan of achieving impressive fitness results, I would like to focus on the subject of positivity. Being positive in everyday life is absolutely huge and is most definitely a game changer. If you can train your mind to always see the positive in any situation and break free of negativity, you will open the gates not only to fitness success but to all types of other advantages in your life in general.

On the example chart in this book, there is a section that is slightly separate. You may want to have a completely separate piece of paper for this but I would advise that you keep your chart as close to a single entity as you can, this way, you are organised and will have a less convoluted view of your chart. So if you do use a separate sheet, you should attach it somehow.

### Filling in your chart

- When it comes to filling in the "5 positive events" section on your chart, you should use events that have happened during your previous week. These don't all have to be fitness related, they could be anything that you have personally recognised as positives over the course of your week. Take a look at the example chart again if you need to. Remember, this is your chart so it's your judgement.

- Make sure that you do this in your first week. This may very well be on the eve of your first training day or before you have even started, but it is a great exercise and measure of your current level of positivity. It may be hard now, but it will be extremely liberating to look back on in six weeks' time and recognise the extent of the development of your mental attitude.

- When you are done filling in the "5 positive events" part of your chart, you should take at least thirty seconds to acknowledge your reason and visual aid if you have one. While you have positive thoughts and energy running through you, it is a great time to reflect on your reasons and the picture in your "visualisation" section of your chart. Remember why you are doing this and promise that you will keep going. The longer that you stick to your routine and new lifestyle plans, the more progress you will have documented. It is always good to look back and recognise how much you have developed. The longer you are in the game, the more impressive your results will be.

### Everyday awareness

Building and strengthening your mental robustness is an ongoing project, just as developing your physical fitness is. If you are a negative person already, you may find that identifying five instances of positive encounters in a week is a hard task. But if you are actively seeking out positive occurrences throughout the week, you will soon find that five examples aren't enough and you can maybe lengthen your quota to ten.

This is why I have added an extra bit to this step. Here is a list of actions that you can easily work on during your everyday life. At work, at home and when you are out and about.

- Learn to spot negativity and when you spot it, find a positive. Everybody has a negative streak to them, but some more than others. Look out for situations in everyday life that show negativity. It may be a close friend or family member that tells you to be less ambitious, it may be a work colleague voicing a negative opinion at a meeting or you may even recognise yourself spouting negativity. As soon as you actively identify your first situation, you will start to see it a lot more frequently.

- When you do encounter an instance of negativity, you should always find a positive counteraction. However dire the situation is, there are always positives.

- If you are in doubt about positivity and mental robustness, you can refresh your memory with the chapter; "Mental challenges" for a reminder of how important mental strength can be.

# Step 4 change & habits

If you want to earn results from a fitness routine. It means that you will be working towards something that you don't already have, and to bring about results, you have to make changes.

The bottom line is that whether you like it or not, your body's physical state is a product of your ongoing habits and lifestyle choices. This means that if you are not 100% happy with your fitness level or your body's physical appearance in regard to the variables that you have control over such as body fat percentage, muscle mass, etc. Then you need to look at what the cause of your discontent is and address it.

Step 4 is about making regular small changes over a period of time and it fits in really well on your chart. The idea is to make one or two changes per week. This means that you will be able to focus on one thing at a time. The longer that you make these changes for, the more changes you will be benefitting from.

**Filling in your wall chart**

- The first thing to do is to identify any bad habits that you have. You should use a notepad to draft these ideas on. The more bad habits you can list or changes that you would like to make, the better. These should be specific changes, the more general the changes are, the harder they will be to initiate or keep track of. For example; if you want to start eating a healthier diet, you should not just write down "eat more healthy food". You should make it specific; you can work on creating a healthy diet over several weeks. An example for a single change in the healthy diet area would be "eat at least one portion of spinach every day".

- Once you have a good sized list of changes (ideally at least ten) you should decide on how many changes you would like to implement each week. I would suggest at least one, but no more than two. It may feel like a great idea to get all these changes done as soon as possible, but in reality, this will put more strain on you need. Remember that the idea is small, focused changes over time. This will result in big

95

changes overall.

- Decide on which changes or habits are most important to you and number them. Once this is done, you should write them on your final chart in the corresponding weeks. These changes and habit substitutions are now official. You should fill in the chart for the coming six weeks at least.

- After each week passes, you should put a big tick over the habit that you changed. If you did not do it, you should strike through it. If for any reason you do not stick to this habit change, carry on with the previous weeks change but do not neglect the new one that you should be focusing on in the coming week. This way, you will always be progressing and a little bump in the road should not force you to start your journey from the beginning again.

# Step 5 Train Smart

Deciding to follow an exercise routine is one thing, but picking a routine that works to most efficiently help you to achieve your fitness goals is another. It is all too common for me to have a conversation with a beginner to fitness about their training requirements and the goals that they want to reach. I am often told that all they want to do is lose weight so there is no need for a resistance exercise programme or weight training routine of any kind.

I always feel like a broken record when I have to explain that an aspect of resistance training should always be incorporated into any balanced exercise routine. By targeting the major muscles of the body with regular resistance exercises will help to build and tone muscle, help with posture, circulation, and fat loss to name a few of the many benefits. And to make your workouts as efficient as they can be, or to put it another way, get the most for your efforts, you should never neglect the resistance side of things, especially if your goal is to lower your body fat percentage.

Having a mix of cardiovascular training (walking, jogging, biking, rowing etc) and resistance training (lifting barbells and dumbbells, using exercise bands and bodyweight exercises etc) is not the only thing that you should look for in a fitness routine. Here is a list of components that in my opinion make an efficient training routine that will give you good results if you are consistent in completing your sessions:

- A good training routine should have some form of cardiovascular training and also some form of resistance training.

- It should be progressive. This means that the exercises should have more than one "upgrade" i.e. it should be progressive in nature, have targets to hit and have several a week timescale. This progression will keep you moving forward and give you a chance to plan out your subsequent weeks of training.

- It should be sustainable. This means that you should be able to continue it for the foreseeable future and build on the basic routine.

- It should take a holistic view and not just target one area of the body. Routines that are set to target "abs", "bums and tums", "biceps" or any other body part alone are what I would call "ancillary workouts". They may be good for the muscle group in question, but they should be viewed as routines that can be used alongside a more substantial training programme.

- If you would like some inspiration or need a solid training routine to get ideas from or to follow completely, I have written several of these for different training goals. So if you would like to jump right in and get started with one of these, you can have a look to see if any would suite you by going to JimsHealthAndMuscle.com. I'll see you there!

## Filling in your wall chart

- Pick the right routine for you. Make sure that you have a good routine that adheres to the criteria above. Again, feel free to check out my website to see if there is something for you.

- Decide when your training days will be each week. I would suggest training at least three times per week on the same day and time. Once you have sorted this out, you should write these days down on your wall chart. Make sure that you fill these days in on your chart for at least six weeks in advance, this way you can tick them off as you go, you will also be able to monitor your progress and have a form of accountability. Make sure to book out time in your diary or schedule for your training. Treat this with the importance of a business meeting, dental appointment or even court summons. There is always time! If you are reading this and feeling unconvinced, please revisit the *"excuses excuses"* chapter for a refresher.

- After each training session, Tick it off, highlight it with a bright marker, stick a gold star or smiley face sticker over it, just mark sure that you mark it in some way that stands out brightly and positively, if you miss a training session for whatever reason, mark it off with a dark colour or a strike through.

# Reward yourself

If you are making big changes to your lifestyle in order to earn fitness success, it can be very hard and feel like you are sacrificing an awful lot. The newer you are to healthy living and fitness training, the harder it will be. For instance, one of the more common reasons for a healthy dieting failure is the thought of never being able to eat your favourite foods ever again.

I can totally empathise with this. I have always had a big appetite and when it comes to pizza, burgers, cheese, chocolate and all of the take away foods that you would associate with unhealthy living, I would be at the front of the queue every time if you could eat this type of food whilst maintaining a good fitness level and physique. When I get invited out for a few drinks with the guys on occasion, I will also be the first there drinking beer and the last to finish on an all-day drinking session.

This may make me sound like a raving alcoholic with an eating disorder and also paint me as a total hypocrite, but the facts are that you do not need to give up everything that you enjoy. You just need to moderate it.

Food is one of my weaknesses but I have managed to get into a good routine of having a cheat meal once per week. Every Saturday night, my girlfriend and I order a takeaway, put on a movie and eat all of the "good stuff" even throwing in, cakes chocolate or other "stickie's" for dessert. So every Saturday night is a night to look forward to and I can tell you that if you are a fast food or chocolate lover and you work hard in staying away throughout the week, when it comes to "cheat night", that food never tasted so good. It is always the best food you have ever eaten which makes it more than worth the wait.

Not everyone is driven by food though, some might like to do a lot of clothes shopping online, have a bottle of wine or a few beers, have a massage or play computer games. The value of a reward can best be determined by the trainer themselves.

### Filling in your wall chart

- Make a list of all of the things that you enjoy doing that have potential to hold you back, ruin your fitness efforts or cost you dearly in some other way ie, if you quit this, it would save you money, time and it does not really offer any real value to your lifestyle.

- Decide if you would like to cut them out completely or start to work on moderating these activities. Once you have decided on which activities you would like to use as your rewards, you can then decide how to fit them in to your new lifestyle.

- In the rewards column on your wall chart, fill in your chosen reward for the completion of each weeks' training, this can be the same every week or you can decide to increase the value of the reward the further that you get into your training. This way, the longer you stay in the game, the better the rewards will be. Another way to fill this in is to have small rewards on a daily basis. For example, if your rewards are diet related, you could have one 100 calorie treat at the end of the day. Obviously a large stuffed crust pizza with extra cheese and garlic bread every day for keeping on track is not a great way to go about rewarding yourself, so be sensible if you go down this route. Personally, I have the same reward every week and one cheat night every week works well for me. This was hard at first but after a month or two, I was able to cope a lot better and even after a few years of this, the novelty has not worn off.

- It is a good idea to fill in the "rewards" section of your wall chart for at least the next six weeks. This way you are planning ahead and once you have reached a reward, tick it off, highlight it in bright colours or use your golden star stickers to make it stand out.

# When it gets tough... And it will get tough.

Things will almost definitely get tough! It might be in your first week, it might be in your third, but everyone struggles at times. If this is the first time that you have tried to stick to a diet plan, fitness routine, or lifestyle change, I can tell you that it will get you down at some stage and you will feel like cheating on your diet, skipping a workout or buying those cigarettes that you have done so well without for the last week or so.

I am no stranger to this place and if there is one thing that has made it increasingly easier for me to stick to my fitness plans over the years when the urges to cheat on my diet or miss a workout is the crushing feeling that I got when I did cave in and eat a bunch of chocolate or miss my workout. It is never worth it. The second I'd finished the "cheat chocolate bar", nothing was any better. The only thing that was different was that my clean record had a blemish on it and that could not be undone. Now the clean record was no longer clean, I may as well make the cheat count, so I would go all in and get more chocolate or junk food. In reality, one chocolate bar is not going to break the bank and I believe that a small slip like this can result in an "in for a penny in for a pound" attitude with most people.

This may be a lesson that has to be personally learned before being fully appreciated, so if you do find yourself in this situation, please remember not to "go all in". A great way to look at it is like this:

If you looked at your day as a percentage and you were good up until you cracked and ate the chocolate bar, it's not a massive loss because you could still finish the day at 90% good. But if you decided to go all in because you believe that all is lost, you could end up having a day that was 90% bad and that is not where you want to be. Remember to be positive!

The main reason for the wall chart is to keep you on track, and if you make this your own, you should use it to draw support from. When you struggle, you might want to go and study it.

- Look at your reason and remember why you are doing this
- Visualise yourself achieving your goal
- Look at motivational quotes.

- The glass is half full! Read your positive experiences
- Look at your progress

The very concept of creating a wall chart may sound silly and sitting in front of it to study it may sound even sillier but believe me, the more work that you put in to this and the more seriously that you approach it, the better that your chances will be. Do not underestimate the power that a physical, visual progression document can have on the outcome of your fitness and lifestyle goals.

# Final Thoughts

There is a lot of information to take in in this book, and I fully understand that many people that read this will decide not to take the time to create a wall chart or any other form of fitness monitoring and tracking system as it may seem like a lot of pointless work and will not feel like it will help towards the final fitness goal.

But any type of fitness goal that is worth earning is not easy work and any edge that you can utilise is worth the time. This is especially true when it comes to developing a solid foundation for your plans. Mind-set plays an extremely important part in your success, so do not neglect this if you really do want some jaw dropping fitness results.

I would like to wish you the best of luck with your health and fitness endeavours and please remember that I would be happy to help you out where I can, so if you have any questions or need some further pointers, I would be glad to help you, please don't hesitate to contact me through one of my websites or social media channels and I will be more than happy to give any advice that I can.

I hope that this has been useful to you and I look forward to hearing of your success and remember if you are looking for a home workout video course to follow as a result of reading this book, please check out the one that I have made!

Whether you chose to invest in this or not, you can still make use of the planning and prep module. This is free to you! So check it out at **YourFitnessSuccess.com** It would be awesome to see you there! ☺

All the best

Jim

(James Atkinson)

If you enjoyed this book, you may also like....

I would like to thank you for reading and again wish you every success with your future fitness plans, whatever they may be. I will also leave you with an excerpt from one of my other books that you may find will compliment this and help you develop your training. This is all about "supersets"

*Excerpt from Jim's weight training guide "Superset style"*

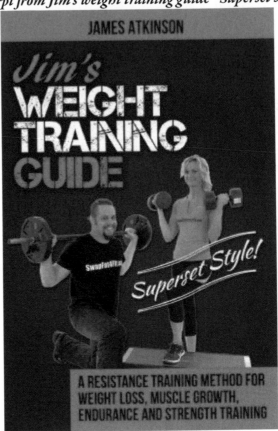

HOW TO GET THE MOST OUT OF THIS BOOK

Because there are many different ways to train with resistance exercise and there are many different goals that can be aspired to, i.e. bodybuilding, endurance, fat loss, etc., the full contents of this book may not be relevant to everyone.

If you are looking for ideas to use superset training to attain results in different areas of fitness, the full content will be useful; but if you are looking for ideas on using superset training for the area of fitness that you are currently involved with, you will probably be able to skip a few chunks of content and revisit it again if you change your fitness goals at a later date.

The book has been split into four sections:

**Section 1:** Covers some of the fundamentals in resistance training. These fundamentals are not only relevant to superset training but they will serve as a solid foundation on which to build any resistance workout routine. Some of this information may also be a nice memory refresher to the basic principles behind weight training for the veteran.

**Section 2:** Covers a selection of example superset workout routines that can be followed directly from the book or modified to suit your personal needs / goals. Some of these example routines may not be relevant to everyone. If you are not interested in some of the training effects outlined, skipping past this information is not a big deal, although it might be useful to see how supersets are employed in different training situations. This might give you some ideas when it comes to designing your own bespoke training plan.

**Section 3:** Gives you all of the information that you need to start planning your own superset training plan. If you wish to follow one of the workout plans that were covered in the previous section, feel free to skip this section. I would advise, however, that you do take a look as there may be something in here that will encourage you to modify your workout plan to make it a bit more bespoke. Even a few little tweaks here and there can make a big difference in the long run.

**Section 4:** This is the section with the exercise descriptions. All of the exercises that are mentioned in the example workout routines are illustrated here. Each exercise description has at least two clear studio quality photographs showing the various stages of the exercise, along with a written account of how to perform the movement safely and correctly. Please have a look at these, even if you normally use these exercises on a regular basis already. We are all guilty of falling into bad habits when it comes to exercise form, and I believe that performing any resistance exercise correctly is one of the top priorities of any workout routine.

INTRODUCTION: WHAT ARE SUPERSETS?

Shortly after the creation of fire but before man invented the wheel, there was a clever little training method developed that was called "Supersets".

As you can see from this brief but accurate account of the origin of supersets, this manner of fitness training has been around for a long time. Like everything else in life, when something has been around for a while, it tends to develop and evolve — and superset training is no exception to this rule.

I have seen superset exercises used in all types of training by all types of trainers and gym rats alike. But due to the lack of structure in this training, I have noticed that, on many occasions, the result or training effect would be far from optimal.

In other words: Why bother training in a certain way if it's not really going to make a difference?

First things first; what is superset training? In the simplest terms, superset training is:

"A sequence of two exercises performed directly after each other with no rest."

It is fairly safe to say that a huge percentage of the population that has trained or looked at examples of different fitness routines will be familiar with the concept of superset training.

But I know from experience that a huge proportion of these guys will not know how to utilise the superset method of training to its full potential. It seems that the usual approach to using superset training is to randomly throw it in on certain muscle groups and training days.

# Connect with Jim

Thank you very much for taking the time to read this section.

I really hope that it has helped you and has given you some ideas on where and how to start with your fitness, lifestyle goals.

Don't forget to visit JimsHealthAndMuscle.com for free fitness, diet and training advice.

If you have any questions or comments, please contact me, Il do my best to help you out.

Like us at Facebook.com/JimsHealthAndMuscle

And follow me on twitter @jimshm

*Other books by James Atkinson*

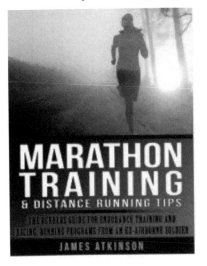

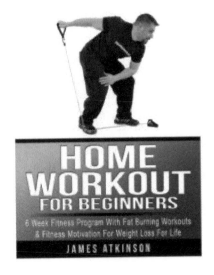

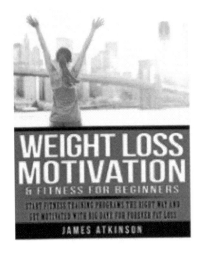

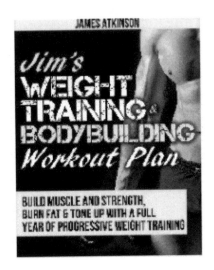

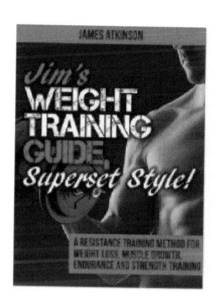

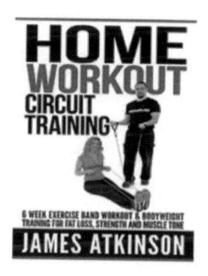

Visit my blog for more great advice on diet,
training, healthy recipes, motivation and more
www.jimshealthandmuscle.com[1]
Please also "Like" and get regular updates on my
Facebook page www.facebook.com/
jimshealthandmuscle
And Follow on Twitter :
@jimshm

---

1. http://www.jimshealthandmuscle.com/

Printed in Great Britain
by Amazon